Technical Manual }
No. 8–215 }

HEADQUARTERS
DEPARTMENT OF THE ARMY
Washington, D. C., *30 April 1969*

NUCLEAR HANDBOOK FOR MEDICAL SERVICE PERSONNEL

CHAPTER 1

INTRODUCTION

1. Purpose

This manual provides a concise reference on nuclear weapons effects of interest to Army Medical Service personnel. It is intended that this information will assist the officers of the Army Medical Department in the conduct of medical service operations in conditions expected in nuclear warfare.

2. Scope

a. The physical characteristics of nuclear weapon detonations and the biological effects which result; principles of diagnosis and management of patients with radiation injury alone or in combination with other injuries; operational problems in areas contaminated by fallout, and medical aspects of nuclear accidents involving nuclear weapons are covered in this manual. Although combat zone nuclear medical and operational problems are emphasized, the basic principles and procedures discussed are also applicable to noncombat zone operations.

b. This manual should be used with other pertinent field manuals and publications. Appendix A lists supplementary references.

c. Users of this manual are encouraged to recommend changes. Comments should be keyed to the specific page, paragraph, and line of the text for which the change is recommended. Reasons for each change should be provided to insure understanding and complete evaluation. Comments should be sent direct to The Surgeon General, ATTN: MEDPT–TO, Department of the Army, Washington, D. C., 20315.

3. Medical and Operational Problems in Nuclear Warfare

a. *Medical Problems.*

(1) *Blast injury.* Blast injuries, such as fractures, lacerations, and puncture wounds, caused by flying debris, displacement, and collapsing buildings are similar for nuclear and conventional weapons. Many of these injuries will be of the type which require immediate attention, notably hemorrhage control, splinting, and dress-ings. These can be performed by nonmedical personnel. The potential patient load and the limited medical means make it essential that commanders place great stress on first aid training.

(2) *Thermal injury.* Large numbers of burns among military personnel are uncommon in conventional warfare in a theater of operations, although burns have occurred in large numbers among civilian populations as the result of non-nuclear, incendiary attacks on cities. With the use of nuclear weapons, however, burns could become one of the most frequent injuries among troops and, as such, constitute the most serious medical problem because of the tremendous logistical requirements associated with adequate burn treatment. The burn victim requires not only extensive support, but highly skilled therapeutic and reconstructive measures as well.

(3) *Radiation injury.* Combat casualties produced by ionizing radiation alone or in conjunction with other injuries or diseases are unique to nuclear warfare. When combined with other injuries, radiation injury will complicate patient management and may increase morbidity and mortality. Radiation injury can occur as a result of a single exposure at the time of a weapon's detonation, exposure to fallout, or from repeated exposures with accumulation of damage.

(4) *Sorting.* Under the conditions of active nuclear warfare, situations resulting in a large number of patients within a short period of time can be anticipated. In such situations, sorting and classification of the patients, necesary at all times in medical operations, becomes critical in order to effectively use the medical means available. The greatest possible number of lives can be saved only by insuring that time and available materials are not expended in heroic but fruitless efforts to save hopeless cases on one hand or in treating patients whose conditions are so minor or uncomplicated that postponement of definitive care is justifiable.

(5) *Radiologically contaminated patients.* Definitive plans and standardized procedures for handling the radiologically contaminated patient

must be developed to minimize the hazard not only to the patient himself, but to the medical personnel who handle or treat the patient. The radiological contamination of patients must not be allowed to interfere with the best possible medical care of these patients.

(6) *Care of civilian patients.* Large numbers of civilian casualties can be expected in nuclear warfare. Consideration must be given to providing, to the maximum extent practicable, emergency medical care and treatment to these civilian patients.

b. Operation Problems.

(1) *Time lag.* Nuclear warfare is likely to increase the time lag between time of injury and time of arrival at the first medical facility. Survivors who eventually reach a medical facility will experience greater morbidity and mortality than similar patients in conventional warfare due to the delay in evacuation and treatment.

(2) *Fallout.* Persistent large area fallout contamination will not only produce its own casualties but at the same time will interfere with medical operations by making movement of patients difficult or impossible. Likewise, the staff of hospitals will be forced to curtail normal operations and seek shelter for an indefinite period.

(3) *Command decisions.* Unique command problems will be encountered in fallout. The medical unit commander must weigh the relative importance of accepting radiation exposure and perhaps casualties in order to accomplish his mission, versus adopting countermeasures against radiation which will reduce this hazard but which may also reduce his immediate operational effectiveness. To make correct decisions and to take effective countermeasures against the hazards of radioactive fallout, the unit commander needs—

(*a*) A local monitoring capability to provide the input data needed.

(*b*) The means of making rapid estimates of future dose and dose rates in a fallout field.

(*c*) Adequate communications to permit rapid reporting of his fallout situation to higher headquarters, and to insure prompt receipt of fallout warnings, information, guidance and orders.

(4) *First aid and rescue.* In the event of mass casualties it is essential that medical service personnel be used primarily in medical facilities to render emergency medical care and treatment and not for first aid or rescue operations.

4. Characteristics of Nuclear Explosions

a. A nuclear explosion is the result of a fission or fusion reaction in which matter is converted into energy. The energy released (the yield of the weapon) is expressed in thousands of tons of TNT equivalent (kiloton or KT), or in millions of tons of TNT equivalent (megaton or MT).

b. As a result of this sudden release of an immense quantity of energy, a fireball is formed which is many times more brilliant than the sun at noon and with temperatures estimated to be of several tens of million of degrees centigrade. The fireball grows in size rapidly, rises like a hot balloon, and cools. The vapors condense to form the mushroom cloud.

c. All energy from the detonation of the weapon is released in three distinct forms: blast, thermal radiation, and nuclear ionizing radiation. The distribution of the energy depends on the nature of the weapon and particularly on the environment of the explosion. At an altitude below 30,000 meters, (100,000 ft) it is generally as follows:

(1) Fifty percent as kinetic energy, which is in the form of a severe blast or shock wave in air.

(2) Thirty-five percent as thermal radiation, which includes infrared, visible light, ultraviolet and some long wave length, soft X-rays.

(3) Fifteen percent as nuclear radiation, which is further subdivided into the following:

(*a*) Five percent initial or prompt radiation, defined as that ionizing radiation emitted during the first minute after detonation.

(*b*) Ten percent residual radiation, defined as that ionizing radiation emitted after the first minute and associated with neutron-induced activity and local/worldwide fallout. Local fallout is defined, somewhat arbitrarily, as those radioactive particles which reach the earth within 24 hours after a nuclear explosion and within several hundred kilometers (or miles) of ground zero. Worldwide fallout consists of smaller particles which ascend into the upper troposphere and into the stratosphere and are carried by the winds to all parts of the earth. It is deposited on the ground over extended periods ranging from months to years.

(4) A diagram of the energy distribution is shown in figure 1.

d. The total amount of energy produced depends on the yield; however, the amount reaching a given target depends also on other factors such as meteorological conditions and the location of the burst with relation to the ground. Bursts are generally classified as follows:

(1) *Airburst*—An explosion in the air above land or water at a height greater than the maximum radius of the fireball. After such a burst, blast may cause considerable structural damage. Burns to exposed skin may be produced over many square kilometers (or miles) and eye injury

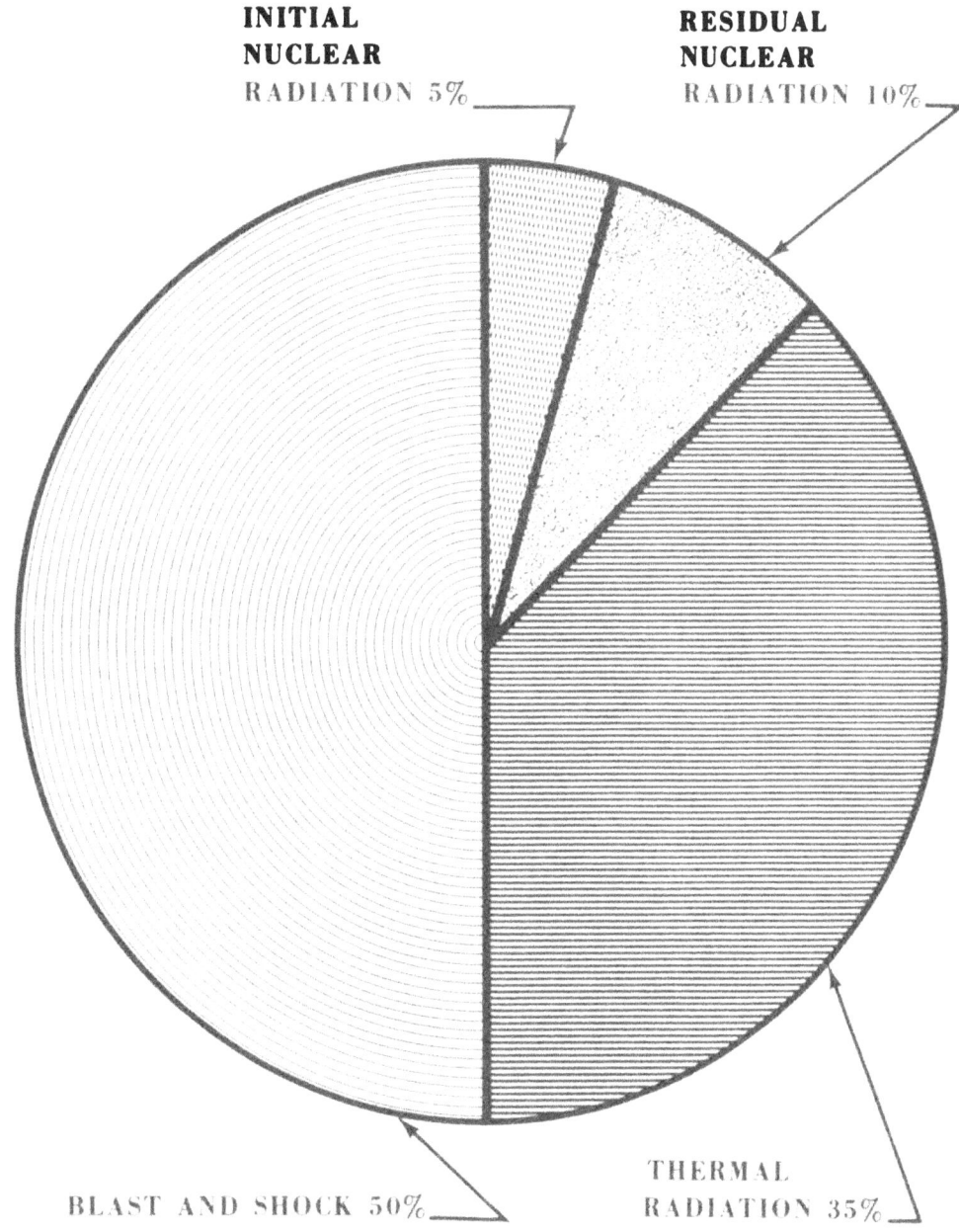

INITIAL NUCLEAR RADIATION 5%

RESIDUAL NUCLEAR RADIATION 10%

BLAST AND SHOCK 50%

THERMAL RADIATION 35%

Figure 1. Distribution of energy

over a still larger area. Initial nuclear radiation will be a hazard at closer distances. The fallout hazard will be negligible. There may be in the vicinity of ground zero an area of induced radioactivity that will be of concern to dismounted troops who may be required to pass through the area.

(2) *Surface or near surface burst*—An explosion at or near the surface of land or water at a height less than the maximum fireball radius. Under this burst condition, the effects of blast, thermal radiation, and initial nuclear radiation will be less extensive than for an airburst of similar energy yield, except in the region close to ground zero where destruction is virtually complete. Local fallout will be a very serious hazard over a very much larger area than that which is

affected by blast and thermal radiation. Induced radioactivity is about the same as in an airburst but is masked by residual radiation from fallout.

(3) *Subsurface burst*—An explosion with its center beneath the surface of land or water. If the burst does not penetrate up out of the surface, the only hazard will be from ground or water shock—no other effects will be significant. If the burst does penetrate the surface (shallow underground burst), the blast, thermal radiation and initial nuclear radiation effects will occur but will be less than for a ground surface burst of comparable yield. Local fallout will also be significant if the burst penetrates up out of the surface.

e. Each form of energy released produces characteristic injuries which will be discussed in detail in the succeeding chapters.

CHAPTER 2

BLAST

5. Physical Characteristics

a. General. After a nuclear detonation, the tremendous quantity of energy released causes a considerable increase in the temperature of all materials in the immediate environment. These materials are converted into gases at very high temperatures and pressures. These gases expand rapidly, pushing away the surrounding air, ground, or water with great force, initiating a blast or shock wave. This wave, moving at high velocity (initially somewhat greater than the speed of sound) expands spherically from the point of detonation, and is responsible for much of the destructive effects of the explosion. Except for subsurface transmission, the wave consists of a thin shell of dense air across which a sharp pressure gradient exists, (from atmospheric pressure (14.7 pounds per square inch at sea level) on the undisturbed side to its peak (known as the peak overpressure)). The fall off back to atmospheric pressure on the inside of the wave is relatively gradual, but very much a function of explosive yield, and is associated with severe displacement of air; this comprises the positive "blast wind." The peak overpressure produces damage to a hollow object such as a building by crushing it, unless the object is strong enough to resist, or unless the object can rapidly reach pressure equilibrium with the overpressure. If the object is elastic, it will resist crushing much more readily than will a rigid structure. The majority of rigid structures will suffer some damage from airblast when the peak overpressure in the blast wave is about 0.5 pound per square inch (psi) or more (shatter glass windows). Five psi will completely destroy a two-story brick house of conventional construction. About 22 psi will cause the collapse of foxholes (>50% filling). 18–42 psi will cause severe damage to tanks, depending upon energy yield of explosion.

b. Dynamic Pressure (Blast Winds). The blast wave, in passing through the atmosphere, imparts energy to the surrounding air molecules, setting them in motion in the direction of the shock front. This motion rapidly develops into a severe transient wind which is generally referred to as the blast wind. The blast wind causes damage by displacement, distortion, or by tearing structures apart. Some indication of the corresponding values of overpressure and maximum blast wind velocities are given in table 1.

c. Effects. While the separate intensities and effects of the peak overpressure and dynamic pressure (blast winds) can be measured, they always occur together. For convenience, the biological effects of these two aspects of blast will be discussed separately, although the injuries which result will be mixed.

6. Direct Blast Injury

a. When the human body is exposed to the environmental pressure variation accompanying a blast wave, the wave is transmitted in complex patterns throughout the body but, more important, the body wall is pushed violently inward. As a consequence of this implosive effect, very high transient internal pressures occur. These often exceed the external pressures by considerable amounts. Severe disruptive forces are produced at junctions of tissues of different densities such as bone with soft tissue or in air-containing organs such as the lungs and abdominal viscera. Only for "long" duration typical blast waves is the severity of the injury sustained roughly proportional to the magnitude of the peak overpressure; otherwise, and in addition, the hazard is a function of the duration and the rate and character of the rise of the pressure pulse. In general, except for the ears and sinuses, the human body is far more resistant to direct blast injury than are rigid structures such as buildings.

Table 1. *Relationship Between Overpressure and Maximum Wind Velocity*

Peak overpressure PSI	Wind velocity (kilometers per hour)
30	1078 (670 mph)
10	467 (290 mph)
5	257 (160 mph)
2	113 (70 mph)

b. While eardrum rupture may occur at peak overpressures as low as 5 psi, the best value of the peak overpressure for 50 percent probability of rupture appears to be between 15 and 20 psi. Though painful, eardrum rupture is not serious. However, infection, fracture and displacement of the ossicles, including the foot plate of the stapes, may result in impaired hearing and require specialized treatment.

c. Blast injuries to the chest begin to occur at about 10–12 psi for "long" duration waves. These include bruising of the soft tissues of the chest wall adjacent to the ribs and rupture of small vascular elements of the pulmonary tissue. Rupture of pulmonary vessels is always associated with interstitial hemorrhage and/or bleeding into the airways. Also, the risk of pulmonary edema is considerable and serious. With severe tearing and rupture, air emboli may occur with grave, frequently fatal, cardiac or cerebral complications. Clinical signs of pulmonary injury may be misleadingly mild until heart failure and edema appear; the heart failure and pulmonary edema are the primary treatment problems. Another matter of great importance in combat is that these patients do not tolerate early evacuation well, particularly if much effort on their part is required. They should not be moved more than absolutely necessary until at least 48 hours after injury, and then with considerable caution. Recurring bleeding of the lungs has been observed up to 5 days after exposure and has accompanied other signs of cardiopulmonary malfunction in delayed fatalities.

d. Blast injuries of the abdomen may include rupture of the liver and spleen, and rarely in airblast, perforations of the intestine. Organ perforations, especially the lower ileum, cecum, and colon are much more common in underwater blast. Also, in airblast hemorrhages of the mesentery and gut wall are almost invariably present. Frequently there is abdominal wall rigidity without perforation or hemoperitoneum, and the significance of the signs and symptoms are difficult to assess. Certainly early differentiation of abdominal from thoracic injury will often require clinical judgment of the highest caliber. In fact, many patients may have degrees of both. Good quality X-rays of the abdomen and chest can be of considerable help as can diagnostic paracentesis to establish the presence of a hemoperitoneum. Early surgical exploration of the abdomen is required for adequate evaluation and treatment. Exploration of the thorax is less often required and should be done only when more conservative measures do not control bleeding.

7. Indirect Blast Injury

a. The high winds associated with blast waves can result in injury from secondary missiles (both penetrating and nonpenetrating) or from displacement of the human body resulting in subsequent severe impact or decelerative tumbling. The injuries which result include wounds from "low" velocity missiles of glass, wood, and gravel, and wounds, such as contusions, and fractures, which result from being thrown against an object. In addition, crush injuries from falling debris can occur. These would be particularly common in urban areas. Troops in the open would be less subject to such injuries. Certain kinds of indirect blast injuries such as violent decelerative experiences or sharp blows to the head from blunt debris are known to produce early lethality just as does primary blast injury to the lung. However, the magnitude and severity of indirect hazards are very much dependent on the conditions of exposure, range, burst type and also upon yield. Thus it is difficult to make a generalized comparison. Even so, for the larger yields the indirect blast effects will occur at greater ranges than primary effects and it is likely that the indirect casualties will be much more common than the primary ones. Many of the latter result in fatalities, as was the case in Hiroshima and Nagasaki, and therefore, they do not enter medical channels and in the tabulations available to define casualty types. Figure 2 illustrates one typical type injury that can be expected as a result of the missile hazard. Principles and techniques of emergency care of these injuries can be found in *NATO Handbook—Emergency War Surgery*.

b. Table 2 summarizes these effects, and illustrates the range within which direct and indirect blast injuries could be expected for various weapon yields.

8. Blast Protection

a. On the Battlefield. Foxholes, bunkers, slit trenches, tanks, and armored personnel carriers offer considerable protection against the effects of blast. If caught in the open, dropping to the prone position with the head directly toward or directly away from the explosion significantly decreases the risk of missile and displacement injuries.

b. In Urban Areas. When specially prepared blast resistant shelter is not available, protection should be sought in the basement of the strongest buildings available.

c. Importance of Time. Since the blast wave travels at approximately the speed of sound (initially a little faster), at distances where protection against blast protection may be effective, eva-

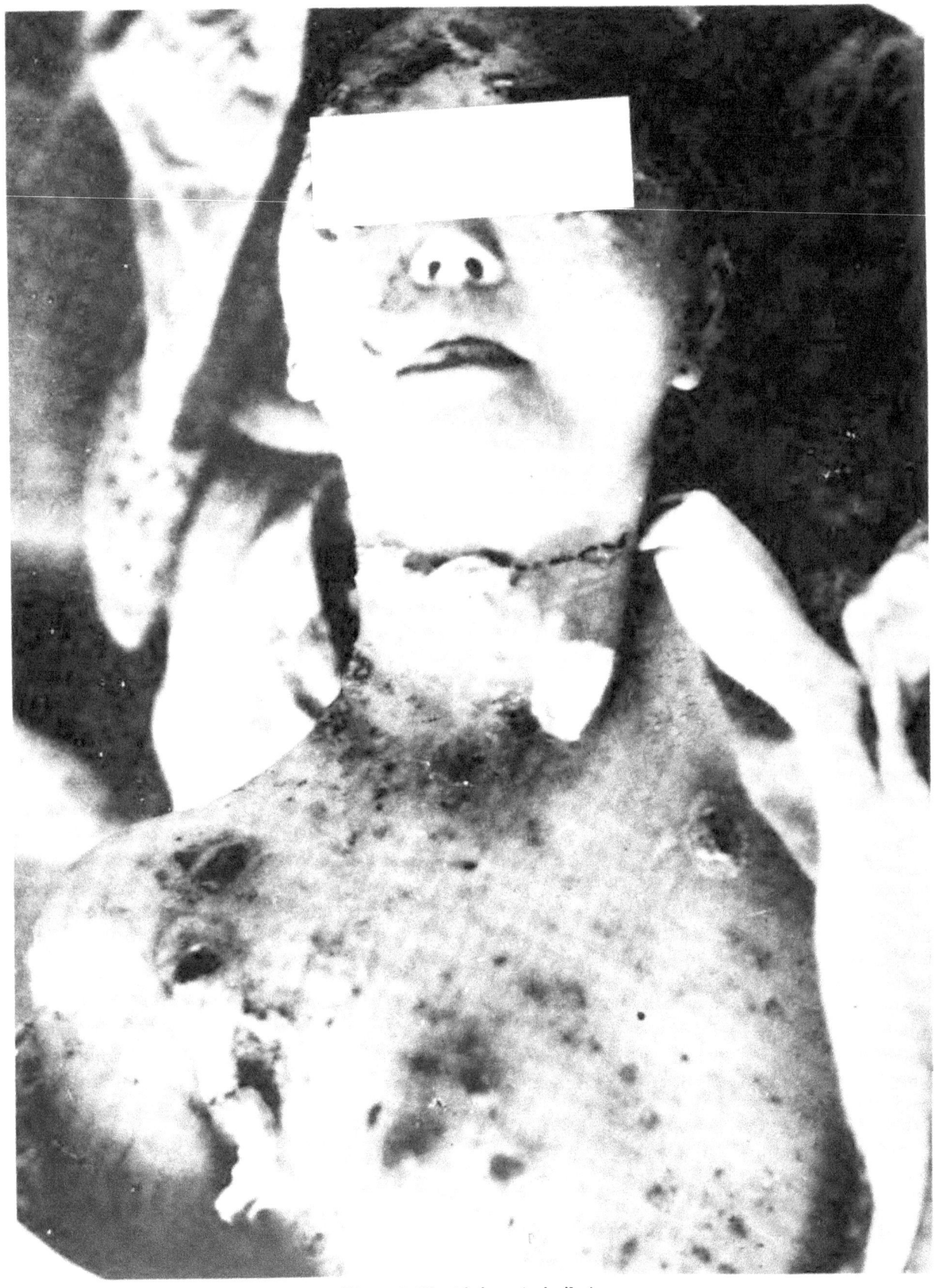

Figure 2. Blast injury (missiles).

Table 2. Tentative Criteria for Production of Direct and Indirect Blast Injuries With Ranges for Various Yield Weapons (Fast Rising, Long Duration Overpressure in Air)

Injury	Peak over-Pressure–PSI	Impact velocity (meters/sec)	Range in kilometers		
			1 KT	10 KT	100 KT
(DIRECT BLAST)					
Eardrum rupture threshold	5	N/A	.7	1.6	3.4
Lung damage threshold	10–12	N/A	.33	.75	1.6
Lethality near 50% probability	42–57	N/A	.16	.35	.76
(PENETRATING MISSILES—10 GRAM GLASS FRAGMENT)*					
Skin laceration threshold	1–2	15 m/sec	1.8	4	9
Serious wound threshold	2–3	30 m/sec	1.2	2.5	5.5
Serious wounds near 50% probability	4–5	55 m/sec	.75	1.8	4
Serious wounds near 100% probability	7–8	90 m/sec	.55	1.3	2.5
(PHYSICAL DISPLACEMENT OF MAN WITH IMPACT WITH HARD SURFACE)*					
Mostly safe (whole body)	3–5	3 m/sec	.75	1.8	4.5
Skull fracture threshold	4–6	4 m/sec	.65	1.6	4
Fractured feet and legs	4–6	4.3 m/sec	.6	1.5	3.6
Skull fracture near 50% probability	5–7	5.5 m/sec	.55	1.4	3.5
Lethality threshold (whole body)	6–8	6 m/sec	.52	1.3	3.1
Skull fracture near 100% probability	6–9	7 m/sec	.49	1.2	3
Lethality near 50% probability (whole-body)	7–10	8 m/sec	.45	1.1	2.8
Lethality near 100% probability (whole-body)	8–11	9.1 m/sec	.4	1	2.5

* In 3 meters of travel.

sive action can be taken. Table 3 gives some approximate values for the times which elapse be-

Table 3. Arrival Time for Peak Overpressure

Distance (kilometers)	1 KT	10 KT	100 KT	1 MT
	(Time in seconds)			
1.6 (1 mile)	4.3	3.6	3.7	2.5
3.2 (2 miles)	>9	8.1	7.4	6.5
4.8 (3 miles)	..	>13	12	11
8.0 (5 miles)	..	..	21	20

tween the instant of the explosion and the arrival time of the blast wave at various distances from ground zero for airburst of various energy yields. It can be seen that at 1.6 kilometers (1 mile) from a 10-KT airburst, which is within the area where protection against blast would be effective (4.6 psi) some 3.6 seconds would elapse before arrival of the blast wave. If prompt action is taken, such as dropping to the prone position as mentioned earlier, the probability of serious missile and displacement injuries is significantly reduced.

CHAPTER 3

THERMAL RADIATION

9. General

a. As a result of the high temperatures generated during a nuclear detonation, a large amount of energy is emitted as electromagnetic radiation. Part of this is in the visible light range, the immediate bright flash characteristic of the nuclear weapon. Much of the rest is in the longer wave length, soft X-ray range. The latter radiation is absorbed rapidly in the immediately surrounding atmosphere, super heating it and resulting in the typical fireball. The fireball in turn emits energy in the infrared, visible, and ultraviolet ranges essentially similar to the spectrum of sunlight. Within the first minute of formation of the fireball this output of electromagnetic radiation is quite intense and very hazardous and can result in burns at considerable distances. It is, therefore, termed thermal radiation and is measured in calories per square centimeter of the surface area of the target.

b. Several factors will vary the thermal effects of nuclear weapons.

(1) *Weapon size.* The thermal output or pulse of weapons increases markedly with increasing yield. A comparison of thermal data for several yields based on their ability to produce second degree burns is shown in table 4. From these data it can be seen that the thermal output follows a different time course with different size weapons and as a result, the amount of thermal energy required to produce the same burn will vary. These data show that a more intense (cal/cm²) thermal pulse is required to produce second degree burns with a larger yield weapon than with a smaller yield weapon. The increased thermal energy is required to compensate for the energy lost during the longer duration of the pulse of the higher yield weapon. With the long duration thermal pulse, the skin is able to dissipate much of the incident thermal energy through reflection and convection. For the short duration pulse of the lower yield weapons, there is not as much time for these processes to cool the skin and a much higher percentage of the energy deposited is available to produce the burn. This does not mean that the thermal hazard is less significant for the higher yields. On the contrary, the total thermal energy released during a nuclear detonation increases markedly with yield, and the effects extend over much greater distances. Therefore, although a more intense thermal pulse is required to produce a given degree of burn for a large yield weapon, the effective range to which this level extends is very much greater than the range at which similar burns can be expected from smaller weapons.

(2) *Use of the weapon.* The altitude at which a weapon is detonated will determine what fraction of its output is thermal. In a very high altitude burst there is much less atmosphere to be heated into a fireball and the nature of the electromagnetic output is considerably changed. In a subsurface burst, the thermal output is absorbed within a short distance below the surface, and is not hazardous to personnel.

(3) *Atmospheric conditions.* The degree of visibility markedly alters the ranges at which thermal effects can occur. The ranges in table 4 are under conditions of unlimited visibility. Cloud cover, fog, and rain, all have definite and varying effects.

10. Thermal Radiation Injuries

a. Burns are caused in two ways and are of two types—

(1) *Direct or flash burns, which result from direct exposure to the thermal pulse.* In general only those parts of the body which are uncovered

Table 4. Radiant Exposures Required to Produce Second-Degree Burns as a Function of Total Energy Yield With Ranges

Yield of weapon	1 KT	10 KT	100 KT	1 MT
Range in kilometers for production of second-degree burns on exposed surfaces (airburst).	0.8	2.4	6.4	18
Duration of thermal pulse in seconds.	0.3	1	2.8	9
Cal/cm² required to produce second-degree burns on exposed surfaces.	4	4.3	5	7

will be burned in this manner. Any object between the fireball and the body will shield and protect against the burn. An exception to this is thin dark clothing, drawn tightly against the body. Under the latter condition, the thermal energy is absorbed in the fabric and burns occur due to contact with the hot fabric as shown in figure 3.

(2) *Indirect or flame burns, which result from exposure to fires caused by the thermal output in the environment, and ignition of clothing.* Depending on the number of flammable objects in an environment this can be the predominant cause of burns. This is particularly true for the larger yield weapons, which can result in conflagrations and firestorms over extensive areas.

b. The effects of thermal radiation injury on the eyes fall into two main categories. These are temporary flashblindness and permanent retinal burns.

(1) Flashblindness is caused by the initial brilliant flash of light produced by the nuclear detonation. More light energy is received on the retina than is necessary for image perception, but less than is required for a burn. The result is "bleaching" of the visual pigments and temporary blindness. During daylight hours, flashblindness generally does not persist for more than about 2 minutes, and only those personnel facing the burst are affected. At night when the pupil is dilated for dark adaptation, flashblindness affects almost all personnel in the target area. Partial recovery, such that personnel could function in lighted areas, may be expected within 10 minutes among those facing the burst, and in about 2 to 3 minutes in all others. Some loss of dark adaptation and night vision will persist for longer periods, however, and can seriously reduce combat effectiveness. From 15 to 35 minutes may be required for recovery of night adaptation, depending upon the level of illumination received.

(2) Retinal burns resulting in permanent damage result from the concentration of sufficient direct thermal energy on the retina by the lens. They occur only if the fireball is in the individual's field of vision. Retinal burns may be experienced at distances from the explosion which exceed those for skin burns. Depending upon the intensity of the exposure and to a great extent upon the part of the retina involved, permanent scarring and interference with vision may occur. As a result of accidental exposures retinal burns have been received in humans at distances of 48 kilometers (32 miles) from an explosion of approximately 200 KT. Retinal burns have been produced in animals at distances up to 480 kilometers (300 miles) from high yield weapons. Retinal burns are

a distinct possibility in nuclear warfare, however, the chances are that only a small proportion of individuals would face the explosion in such a way that the fireball would be in their field of vision.

(*a*) Figure 4 illustrates the estimated threshold distances at which flashblindness and retinal burns may occur following airburst of various weapon yields. The following assumptions were made in the preparation of figure 4:

1. Personnel are dark adapted.
2. Exposure to 10^{-4} calories/cm² will produce flashblindness in a dark adapted person.
3. The combination of a retinal exposure of 0.16 calories/cm² and a retinal fireball image of 2 mm will result in a clinically significant retinal burn.
4. Atmospheric transmittance is that of a clear day.

(*b*) A 2-mm diameter lesion was arbitrarily selected as a critical sized injury; however, much smaller lesions could result in serious visual impairment. *For example,* the most serious damage to vision occurs when the fireball is focused on the fovea, which measures 0.44 mm in diameter, since this area is responsible for fine central visual acuity. Less critical but major functional impairment is noted when the macula, which extends to a diameter of 1.7 mm, is affected. On the other hand, a lesion as large as 5 mm in the periphery of the retina would probably cause no functional distress.

(*e*) For airbursts, the range for chorioretinal burns exceeds that of other significant weapons effects only for yields of about 1 kiloton or greater. For surface burst weapons this transition occurs at about 0.1 kiloton. From this we may conclude that chorioretinal burns should not be a tactically significant problem for airbursts of about 1 KT or less, or for surface bursts of about 100 tons or less. For the dark adapted individual, the range for flashblindness exceeds that for chorioretinal burns by a factor of 30 or more.

(3) See table 5 for a summary of the visual effects of nuclear detonation.

11. Classification of Burns

Burns are generally classified according to the depth of the tissue involved.

a. First degree burns, in which the outer layers (epidermis) of the skin are injured but not destroyed, produces only redness of the skin. Second degree burns are deeper, extending into the dermis, and more severe, and are characterized by the formation of blisters. In third degree burns, the full thickness of the skin is involved.

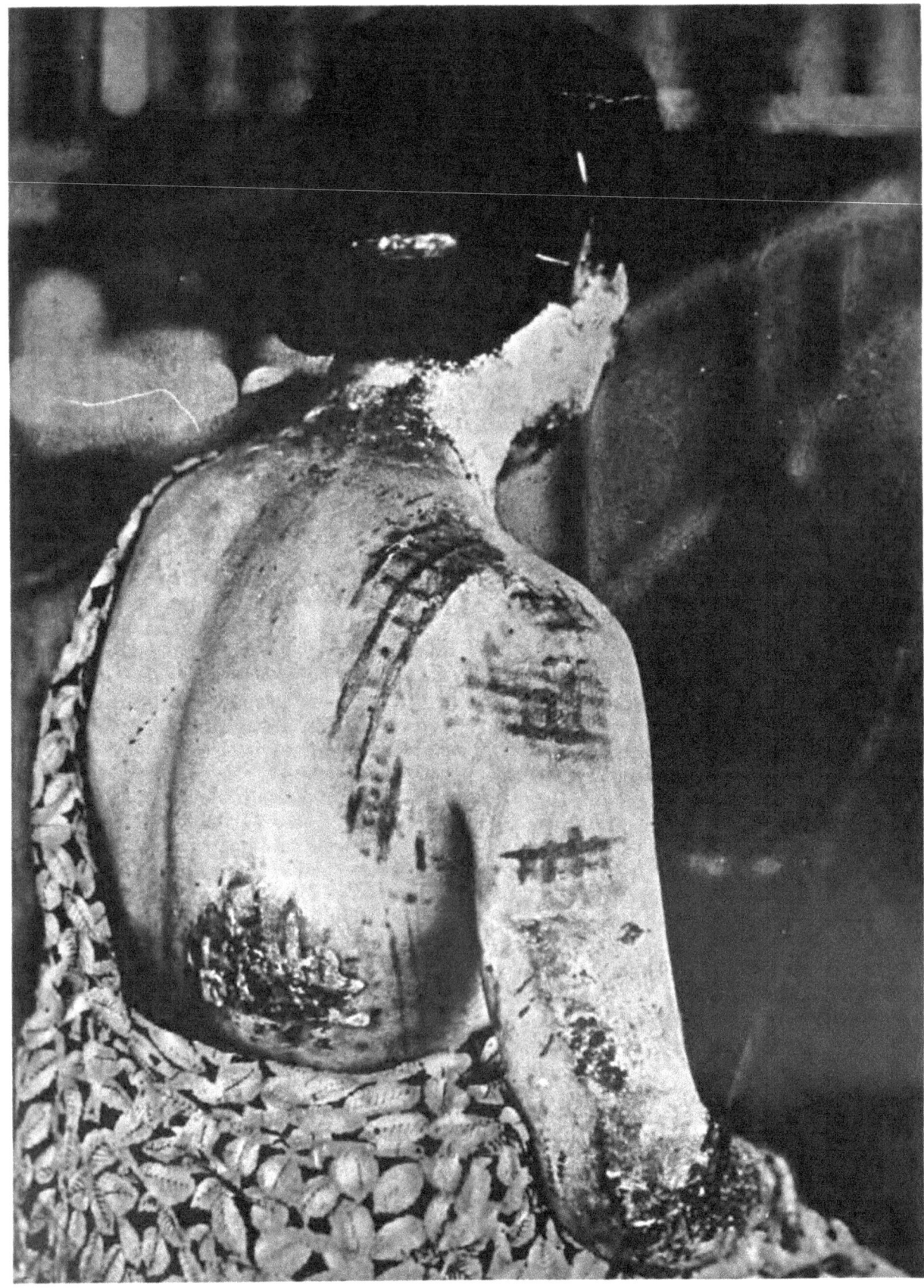

Figure 3. Flash burn through dark clothing.

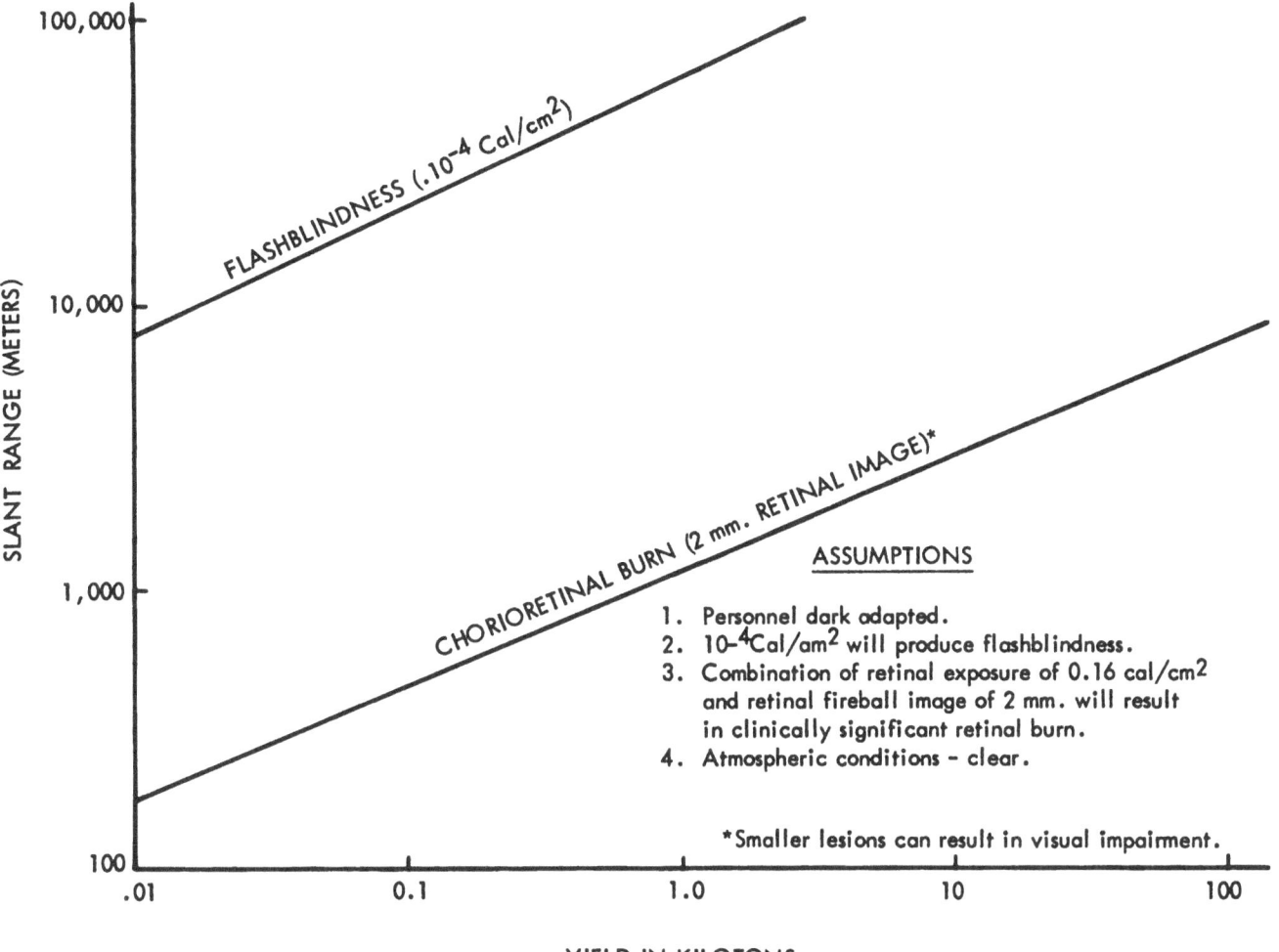

Figure 4. Threshold distance for minimal chorioretinal burn and flashblindness versus yield (airburst).

b. The distribution of burns into these three degrees has certain limitations, as it is not always possible to differentiate between first and second degree or between second and third degree burns.

c. The extent of the area of the skin which has been affected by the burn is a major factor in determining prognosis. A second degree burn over a large area of the body will be more serious than a small third degree burn. However, there are certain critical regions, such as the hands, face, eyes, and genitalia, of which almost any degree of burn will seriously incapacitate the individual.

(1) To estimate the area of a burn injury, the "rule of nines" is useful, inasmuch as it divides the body surface into areas of 9 percent or multiples thereof, as shown in figure 5. This allows rapid estimation of the extent of the body involved, and forms a rational starting point for the planning of treatment.

(2) In young healthy adults, burns of 20 percent or less of the body surface have practically no associated mortality. Burns involving between 20 and 40 percent of the body surface have a slowly rising probability of mortality up to 20 percent. When more than 40 percent of the body surface is burned, the mortality increases abruptly and rapidly as the involved surface increases. With a 60–65 percent body burn there is a 50 percent mortality, whereas there is a 90 percent plus mortality with a 70 percent burn. In addition, morbidity and mortality are increased by thermal injury to the pulmonary tract and by the combination of severe mechanical and/or radiation injury with the burn.

12. Treatment

It should be emphasized again that in usual combat situations burns are uncommon. Therefore, no special planning for the care of large numbers of burned patients is required. In nuclear warfare, this is not true, and consideration must be given to the increased need for medical support which would result from a high incidence of burned patients.

a. In combat, the methods of treatment for burns must be standardized.

Table 5. Summary of Visual Effects of Nuclear Detonation

Time of day	Orientation	Flashblindness	Loss of night adaption	Retinal burns
DAYTIME	1. Eyes focused on point of detonation.	1. Yes: Recovery in approximately 2 minutes.	1. N/A	1. Very likely
	2. Burst in field of vision but not focused on point of burst.	2. Yes: Recovery in less than 2 minutes.	2. N/A	2. Possible
	3. Personnel shielded or looking away.	3. Not very likely	3. N/A	3. No
NIGHTTIME	1. Eyes focused on point of detonation.	1. Yes: Recovery gradual in 10 minutes or less. Will depend upon visual task to be performed and level of illumination.	1. Yes: Recovery gradual in 15 to 35 minutes.	1. Very likely
	2. Burst in field of vision but not focused on point of burst.	2. Yes: Recovery in approximately 5 minutes or less for most situations. Depends upon visual task to be performed and level of illumination.	2. Yes: Recovery gradual in 15 to 35 minutes.	2. Possible
	3. Personnel shielded or looking away.	3. Possible from reflection. Recovery in 2 to 3 minutes for most situations. Depends upon visual task to be performed and level of illumination.	3. Possible: Recovery in no less than 15 minutes.	3. No

(1) A standard fluid therapy formulation, such as the "Brooke Formula," can provide the basis for planning resuscitative fluid therapy. According to this formula, the intravenous fluid requirements during the first 24-hour period are—

(a) Colloids, such as blood, plasma, or plasma expander, 0.5 ml. per kilogram of body weight for each percent of body surface burned up to 50 percent.

(b) Electrolytes, 1.5 ml. per kilogram for each percent of body surface burned up to 50 percent.

(c) Glucose and water, 2,000 ml.
During the second 24 hours, the requirements are usually one-half of the first 24 hours. However, rigid adherence to a treatment plan based on a formula may lead to serious errors in management. Each patient must be followed individually and the fluid replacement adjusted accordingly. The best single guide to the state of hydration is the urinary output, and it should be monitored closely and continuously. Since combat burns are not scald injuries with the attendant marked fluid shifts, overhydration can occur unless the fluid requirements are continuously reevaluated watching for signs of pulmonary edema. Although inadequate fluid replacement is a very serious risk, overzealous fluid therapy can be an equal hazard.

(2) Almost all burns should be covered with dressings. This allows evacuation of patients at any time after the initial 72-hour period of instability is passed. It is also the preferred way to handle burns in makeshift surroundings.

(3) All burns in combat should receive antibiotics during treatment because of the hazard of infectious complications.

b. When the facilities for treating burn patients are limited, consideration may have to be given to the administration of fluids orally, utilizing a formulation such as Haldane's solution. This solution is prepared by dissolving 3 to 4 grams of salt (½ teaspoonful) and 1.5 to 2 grams of bicarbonate of soda (½ teaspoonful) in each quart of water. This can be a most effective method of fluid replacement when the casualty load is excessive, as it does not require skilled nursing personnel. It is ideally suited to the care of patients in isolated units with limited medical facilities, since the material for it could be airdropped. Further, it can and must be started early in order to be effective.

c. Certain burn patients will have a poor prognosis. These include—

(1) Those with extensive, deep burns, second and third degree, over 40 percent or more of the body surface.

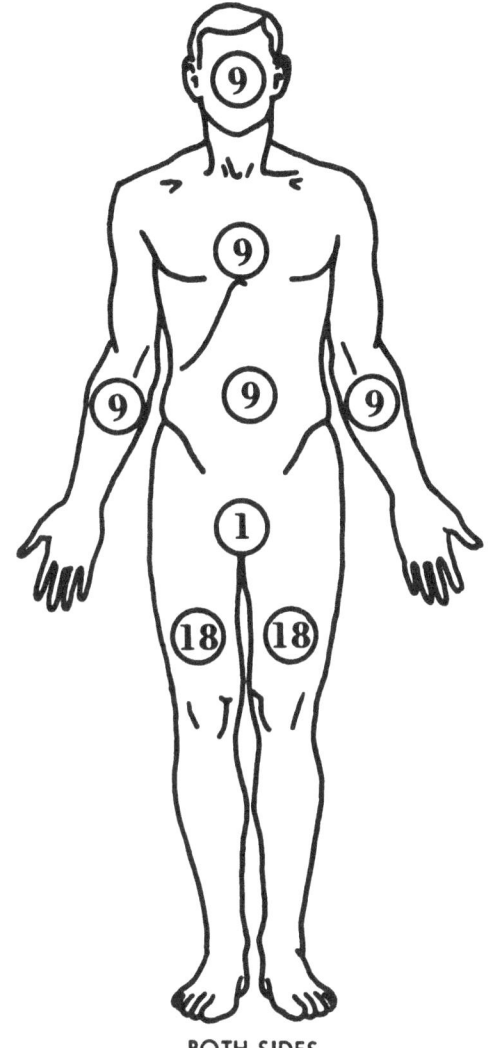

BOTH SIDES

Figure 5. Rule of nines.

(2) Those with deep pulmonary burns. Not all patients with head and neck burns have deep pulmonary burns. Those exposed to direct flash injury only would be unlikely to have sustained a serious pulmonary injury. People caught in flaming surroundings, however, are likely to suffer tracheobronchial burns due to the inhalation of hot gases or aerosols. If the injury is limited to the trachea and main stem bronchi, the patients may well survive, whereas a deep pulmonary injury involving the bronchial tree and alveoli carries with it a high probability of mortality. In the field, early differentiation between nonfatal and fatal pulmonary injuries would be difficult. But, patients with any signs of pulmonary injury, particularly pulmonary edema, probably should be considered as having a poor chance of survival.

d. More detailed consideration of burn injuries may be found in the *NATO Emergency War Surgery Handbook.*

13. Thermal Protection

a. As mentioned earlier, the hazard from thermal effects of nuclear weapons is a function of the intensity and duration of the weapon's thermal output. With increasing weapon yield, the thermal output is more intense and the duration is much longer. In addition, the larger the weapon, the more time it takes for the thermal output to reach its maximum. If caught in the open, evasive action to minimize flash burn injury should be taken if possible before or soon after the thermal maximum is reached since at this time only 20 percent of the thermal energy will have been received. The elapsed times between the instant of explosion and thermal maximum for air and surface bursts of various energy yields are shown in table 6. From this table it can be seen that the prospects of being able to take evasive action are not good for bursts of low energy yield, but some possibility may exist for explosions in the megaton range.

b. At the first indication of a nuclear explosion, by a sudden increase in the general illumination, an individual caught in the open should fall prone to the ground, and if possible, crawl behind a tree, building, fence, ditch, bank, or any structure which prevents a direct line of sight between himself and the fireball. If no substantial object is at hand, the clothed parts of the body should be used to shield parts which are exposed. There will still be some hazard from scattered thermal radiation, especially on a hazy day from high yield weapons at long range, but the decrease in the direct radiation will be substantial.

c. If inside a building a person should immediately fall prone also, and if possible, crawl behind or beneath a table or desk. Even if this action is not taken soon enough to reduce the thermal radiation exposure greatly, it will provide a partial shield against splintered glass and other flying debris and minimize the displacement effect of the blast wave.

d. Clothing of the proper kind provides good protection against flash burns. Materials of light color are usually preferable to dark materials. Woolen materials give better protection than those of cotton of the same color, multilayer garments

Table 6. Time Between Detonation and Maximum Thermal Output

| | Explosion Yield | | | | |
	1 KT	10 KT	100 KT	1 MT	10 MT
Time (seconds)	0.03	0.1	0.3	1.00	3.2

are better than single layer, loose better than tight, and the heavier the fabric, the greater the protection.

e. Protection against eye injury is difficult, especially for those who happen to be facing the burst point. Ordinary sunglasses will provide little or no protection against eye damage. Although there is a low probability that personnel will be looking up at the sky and facing the burst point, the fireball of a high yield weapon detonated within the atmosphere persists for a sufficient duration to attract attention, allow for orientation behavior and fixation, and several eye blinks. Conversely, there is time for the trained individual to initiate protective action (blink and look away) which could save him from serious eye effects. It is doubtful, however, that the same protective measures would be effective at those distances where the same total amount of thermal energy is received from weapons of lower energy.

CHAPTER 4

NUCLEAR RADIATION

14. General

a. *Ionizing Nuclear Radiation.* Ionizing nuclear radiation is a phenomenon entirely different from any encountered with conventional, nonnuclear weapons. It is an additional casualty producing mechanism superimposed on the others already discussed. Ionizing radiation is emitted in various forms with time during and after a nuclear detonation, and as stated earlier has been arbitrarily divided into two categories—

(1) Initial or prompt radiation, which is emitted during the first 60 seconds and which results almost entirely from the nuclear processes in the detonation.

(2) Residual radiation which is emitted after 1 minute and which is derived predominantly from decay processes of isotopes (the fission products) produced during the detonation.

b. *Initial Nuclear Radiation.* During the nuclear detonation, the nuclear material present within the warhead undergoes either fission or fusion reactions resulting in the emission of highly energetic ionizing nuclear radiations. These consist primarily of neutrons and gamma rays and lesser amounts of beta radiation. The neutrons and some of the gamma rays are produced almost instantly by fission and fusion (when a fusion stage is included in the warhead) processes while the remaining gamma radiation and the total beta contribution result from decay of fission products with short half-lives. Alpha radiation is also present and is primarily the product of either the decay of the unfissioned uranium or plutonium or the fusion process when a fusion stage is included in the warhead.

c. *Residual Nuclear Radiation.*

(1) Residual radiation includes neutron-induced radioactivity in the soil and material near the detonation, and fallout, which may be distributed over many square kilometers and at great distances from the point of detonation.

(2) Neutron-induced radioactivity occurs when free neutrons from the detonation interact with elements in the atmosphere and ground in the vicinity of the detonation making them radio-active. Most of these radioactive elements decay rapidly, emitting both gamma and beta radiations. The resulting gamma hazard can be as serious as that due to fallout and can be great enough to deny access to the contaminated area. However, the geographic area in which this induced radioactivity is produced is many times smaller than that usually involved in fallout since it is limited to an area immediately around ground zero.

(3) Fallout is the process in which radioactive material rises with the fireball of a nuclear detonation into the upper atmosphere and then falls back to earth over a variable period of time due to gravity, rain-out, or snow.

(a) Fallout is composed of several different radioactive materials as follows:

1. Unfissioned uranium or plutonium from the weapon.

2. Fission products which are generally elements with atomic weights about $\frac{1}{3}$ to $\frac{2}{3}$ that of uranium or plutonium.

3. Weapon debris, soil, water and other material in which radioactivity has been induced by neutrons.

(b) The particles suspended initially in the rising fireball settle to earth eventually by gravity. The rates and patterns of settling depend upon the yield of the weapon, the height of burst, the particle size distribution, and meteorological conditions.

(4) Fallout in a given area presents three hazards—beta contamination of the skin, irradiation of the body or organs by isotopes taken into the body, and external whole body gamma irradiation.

(a) *Beta contamination of the skin.* This hazard results from the deposition of radioactive fallout material directly upon the unprotected skin. If not removed for several hours, superficial beta skin burns can be produced. Since serious injury would not result from this injury, and prevention is easy, it is considered to be of minor significance in combat operations (para 20).

(b) *Internal hazard.* This hazard results from the retention of radioactive fallout material in the body following inhalation or ingestion, or absorption through wounds. This normally represents a long term hazard and is, therefore, not of immediate importance on the battlefield (para 21).

(c) *External whole-body gamma hazard.* Whole-body gamma irradiation results from the exposure of the individual to penetrating gamma radiation from material dispersed on the ground in an area contaminated by fallout or by neutron-induced radioactivity. It is by far the most important of the three fallout hazards on the nuclear battlefield (para 18).

15. Basic Physical Characteristics of Ionizing Radiation

a. Nuclear Radiations. The four nuclear radiations, alpha particles, beta particles, gamma rays, and neutrons, produce their various biological effects by the same physical process, the transfer of energy to target molecules. The relative biological effect of a given type of radiation depends upon the distribution and the quantity of energy deposited or absorbed in tissues. The radiation dose is defined and described in terms of the amount of energy absorbed per unit mass (para 16). One of the major effects of radiation of any type in tissue is thought to be ionization.[1] Charged particles, alpha and beta, cause a high concentration of ionization by interacting with orbital electrons along their path through matter. Gamma rays ionize occasional atoms along their paths in matter, but the secondary electrons thus produced will in turn ionize densely. Neutrons, being uncharged, produce ionization by interacting with atomic nuclei. They may be captured by nuclei, producing an unstable state and subsequent prompt or delayed radioactive decay or they may collide with nuclei and transfer to them a portion of their kinetic energy. The nuclei will be displaced from their electron shells and, since they are charged, will in turn ionize densely along their short paths. Therefore, there is a basic similarity between these radiations, and they can all be termed "ionizing." Despite the common factor of ionization, the four radiations do have important differences, warranting separate discussion.

b. Alpha Particle. Structurally, the alpha particle is identical with the nucleus of the helium atom. It contains two protons and two neutrons for a total atomic mass of four, with a double positive electrical charge.

(1) Alpha particles are emitted by the *unfissioned* plutonium or uranium of a weapon. They

result from the normal radioactive decay of these substances. Compared to the other forms of radiation, the alpha particle is very heavy, highly charged, and slow. It ionizes very densely in any target material, but it has a very short range. In air it travels about 5 cm. (2–3 inches), but in tissue, a fraction of a millimeter. Because its energy is absorbed by the outermost layer of the skin or even by a thin sheet of paper, alpha particles produce no hazard so long as it remains outside the body.

(2) Inhalation or ingestion, with absorption of alpha emitting isotopes into the body may constitute a long range health hazard in industrial environments or at nuclear weapon accident sites. But significant quantities of such isotopes will not occur in any area in wartime, even though they are present both at the time of detonation and in the fallout associated with ground burst weapons.

c. The Beta Particle. The physical characteristics of the beta particle are the same as those of the orbital electron even though it originates from the nucleus of a radioactive fission product. Most radioactive elements which result from uranium or plutonium fission are beta emitters.

(1) The beta particle is small ($\frac{1}{7400}$ the size of an alpha particle). It may travel initially at speeds up to about 95 percent of the speed of light, and it has a single negative electrical charge. Being charged, small, and fast, it ionizes over greater distances but less intensely than the alpha particle. Its range in air is about 5 meters (15 feet), whereas, in tissue, it is a few millimeters or centimeters, depending on its initial energy.

(2) Beta particles from radioisotopes associated with fallout will penetrate into the superficial cell layers of the skin, producing "beta burns" after prolonged contact. Shielding against beta particles is provided by interposing clothing, canvas, or other easily available material between the source and the skin. Contact beta burns can be reduced or avoided by early brushing or washing fallout material from the surface of the body. Careful troop indoctrination in these simple methods of decontamination of exposed skin surfaces and skin folds will assist in holding beta burns to a minimum. While the military hazard is small compared to gamma radiation, it cannot be ignored.

d. The Gamma Ray. Gamma rays are electromagnetic radiations emitted by the nuclei of some radioactive isotopes. The characteristic features of gamma radiation are its electromagnetic nature and ability to penetrate and ionize many materials. Since it is an electromagnetic radiation,

---

[1] The process whereby energy is acquired by a neutral atom or molecule resulting in the ejection of an orbital electron and producing two charged particles, i.e., an ion pair.

it travels at the speed of light (3×10^{10} cm/sec or 186,000 miles per second).

(1) Gamma radiation of high energy (average: 4 Mev for nuclear weapons) is produced by the process of fission and comprises a large part of the initial radiation. Also, many fission products and their daughter products emit gamma rays, lower in energy (average: 0.7 Mev) than that produced by the fission process. Since gamma rays are not charged particles, they ionize indirectly by producing energetic electrons in the material in which they are absorbed. The energy of these electrons is then dissipated by intense localized interaction with matter. Because the attenuation per unit length of path of the primary gamma ray is relatively small, these secondary electrons may be produced at considerable depth in the target.

(2) As gamma rays pass through tissue, absorption is nearly exponential so that theoretically at least some fraction of the gamma energy will pass through any thickness of the material. Figure 6 shows this absorption for gamma radiation of 1.25 Mev energy (average energy ^{60}Co.). Figure 6 shows that at a depth of 13.6 cm. or about 5 inches about 50 percent of the gamma rays

have been absorbed. This is a highly penetrating form of radiation.

(3) For the low energy (<0.5 Mev) and high energy (>5.0 Mev) gamma rays, dense materials such as lead are more effective absorbers or shields than are those of low atomic weight. For gamma rays with intermediate energy, attenuation or shielding is a function more of thickness of material alone and is practically independent of the kind of material.

(4) Shielding against gamma rays from fallout radiation is of prime importance in military planning. Fortunately, readily available materials such as concrete, earth, steel, and sand in bags, will provide adequate shielding against gamma radiation if used in appropriate thicknesses and its relation to angle of incidence.

e. The Neutron. The neutron is an electrically neutral (uncharged) particle, approximately 1 atomic mass unit in weight. It is a normal constituent of all atomic nuclei except that of the common isotope of hydrogen. It is produced during the fission reaction along with fission products and kinetic energy. Some of the neutrons produced will go on to cause other fission reactions, which

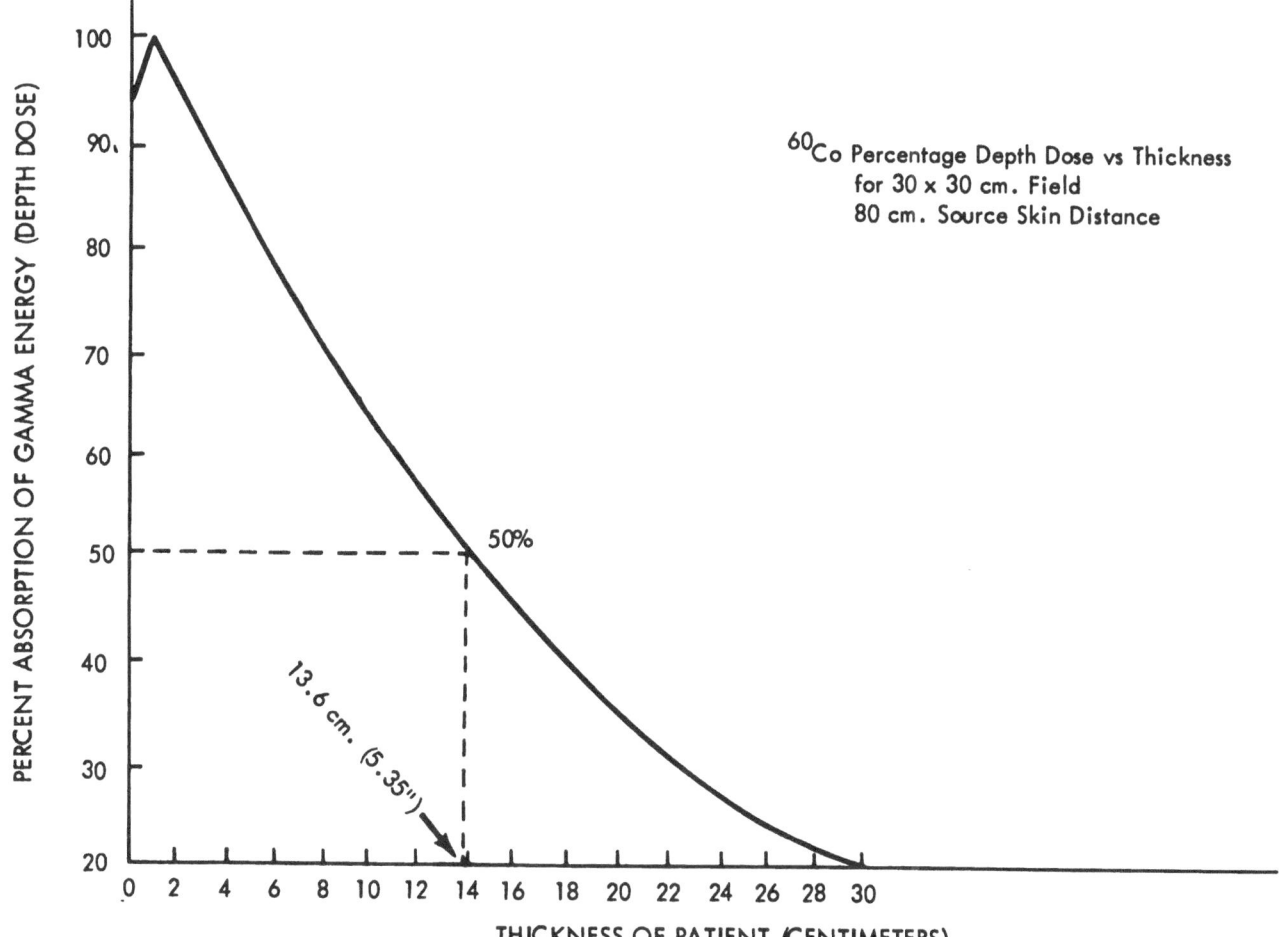

Figure 6. Absorption of gamma energy in tissue.

are necessary to sustain the reaction of a nuclear explosion. Others will be lost to the environment as part of the initial radiation. Fusion of the heavier isotope of hydrogen produces helium, free neutrons, and energy.

(1) Since neutrons are produced in enormous numbers mainly during the actual reactions of fission or fusion, they contribute only to the initial or prompt radiation hazard. Their contribution to the fallout problem can be significant, however, because of their ability to induce certain materials to become radioactive. Nonfissionable portions of the bomb structure, air atoms, and certain elements in soil and water are some of the substances in which radioactivity can be induced. These, with all other materials in the near vicinity of the detonation are vaporized and, after cooling and condensation, become part of fallout.

(2) Since neutrons have no electrical charge, they do not ionize by interaction with orbital electrons. Fast or high energy neutrons, produced during fission or fusion, lose energy to and ionize target atoms primarily by "collision" with the nuclei of those atoms, especially hydrogen. After "collision" the neutrons and the target nuclei (protons in the case of hydrogen) "recoil" in a manner which has been likened to the action of billiard balls. The target protons are stripped of their orbital electrons by this process and are, therefore, ionized. Since they are charged particles, the resulting protons cause dense concentrations of secondary ionizations along their short paths in the target material. Protons ionize more densely than do beta particles and less densely than alpha particles. The protons may be produced at considerable depth in tissue by this collision process. Therefore, fast neutrons qualify as penetrating ionizing radiations, somewhat similar in this respect to gamma radiation.

(3) When the target atoms are heavier than hydrogen, the neutrons lose less energy with each collision. If the target nuclei are quite heavy, essentially no energy is lost by the neutrons, and they are only scattered. Therefore, shielding made of lead or other heavy metals does not significantly impede neutrons although it will scatter them widely.

(4) Very slow, low energy neutrons (the end result of many collisions and termed "thermal neutrons") interact with matter finally by nuclear capture. This can occur with a great variety of target elements, resulting in the formation of unstable, radioactive isotopes. These isotopes in turn emit beta particles and/or gamma rays as they decay.

(5) Whole body radiation injury from neutrons is, about equivalent to that produced by absorption of an equivalent amount of energy from gamma irradiation. However, for specific tissues, for example the lens of the eye or the gastrointestinal mucosa, neutrons are more injurious than are gamma rays of equal absorbed dose. In other words, for certain end results neutrons have a greater relative biological effectiveness (RBE) (para 16c).

(6) It is generally more difficult to shield against neutrons than against gamma rays. The dense materials adequate for protection against gamma radiation may scatter neutrons widely but impede them only slightly. Hydrogenous materials such as water, dirt, and modified concrete are the most effective absorbers of fast neutrons available in the field since there will be considerable transfer of energy to protons during the scattering of the neutrons within the material.

(7) With megaton weapons, defense against neutrons (or prompt gamma) is not necessary since high levels of blast and thermal radiation occur at distances from ground zero far beyond that reached by significant prompt radiation. With low yield tactical weapons, against which defenses from heat and blast are practical, prompt radiation, including the neutron component, may represent a major hazard. The characteristics of the four radiations are summarized in table 7.

16. Units of Measurement and Definitions

Discussion of the biological effects of radiation requires understanding of certain basic terminology.

a. *Roentgen.* This is the basic unit used for quantifying exposure doses of radiation and commonly written as "R." It is limited by definition to ionization produced in air by gamma or X-radiation in the energy range between 30 Kev and 3 Mev. Therefore, so far as man as a target is concerned, roentgens describe an air dose to which he is exposed and not the amount of energy his tissue absorbs. Specifically, one "R" is equivalent to 1.0 electrostatic unit of charge of either sign in 0.001293 grams of air (1.0 cc at 0°C and 760-mm Hg atmospheric pressure) or roughly, one "R" is equal to about 93 ergs of energy per gram of air. The same degree of ionization may be produced in air by radiations which have different energies but the patterns and distribution of ionization in tissue may be quite different. Therefore, one cannot translate directly from an exposure dose in roentgens to an absorbed dose without additional information. Further, the term roentgen cannot be used to describe the dosage, even in air, of particulate radiations, such as neutrons, beta particles, or alpha particles. The com-

Table 7. *Characteristics of Nuclear Weapon Radiations*

NAME AND SYMBOL	WHAT IS IT	SOURCE	ENERGY AND SPEED	RANGE IN AIR	RANGE IN TISSUE	SHIELDING REQUIRED	BIOLOGICAL HAZARD (WARTIME)
α Alpha Particle	Helium Nucleus	Decay of Uranium and Plutonium	Energy varies: speed varies from 1/20 c to 1/10 c	~5 cm⁻	Cannot penetrate the epidermis	None	None, unless ingested or inhaled in sufficient quantities
β Beta Particle	High speed electron	Decay of fission products and neutron induced elements	Varies	5 meters	Several layers of skin	Stopped by a few cm of Al or moderate clothing	Superficial skin injury
γ Gamma Ray	Electromagnetic energy	Decay of fission products and neutron induced elements	Energy varies; travels at the speed of light (c)	Up to 500 meters, but energy dependent	Very penetrating, but energy dependent	Dense material, e.g.—concrete, steel plate, earth	Whole body injury; many casualties possible
n Neutron	Uncharged particle	Fission and fusion reactions	Varies	Less than gamma but energy dependent	Very penetrating, but energy dependent	Hydrogenous materials: e.g. water or damp earth	Whole body injury; many casualties possible

monly used multiple in clinical medicine of the roentgen is the milliroentgen (mr), which is 1/1,000 of a roentgen.

b. Rad. A unit of radiation which expresses the absorbed dose. It represents the deposition of 100 ergs of energy per gram of the target material or tissue. A standard target material is not specified and the same exposure dose in roentgens could easily result in different absorbed doses in rads in different target materials. Conversion from an exposure dose in roentgens to an absorbed dose in rads requires knowledge of the relative patterns of energy deposition in air compared with the material in question. The rad is not limited to ionization as is the roentgen. This is reasonable since ionization is only one of the ways in which radiation energy affect the target atoms and molecules in a solid target such as living tissue. Also, the rad can be applied to any form of electromagnetic or particulate radiation. At present, no field dosimeters measure directly in rads. For field work, the measured exposure dose in roentgens is assumed to be equivalent to the absorbed dose in rads. Errors introduced by this assumption are felt to be small compared with the other sources of errors and the variabilities in response to radiation. FM 101–31–1 directs that the "rad" be used throughout the Army for training and operational purposes. The commonly used multiple is millirad (mrad), which is 1/1,000 of a rad.

c. R.B.E. An abbreviation for Relative Biological Effectiveness. This term, expresed as a number, was designed to allow quantification of the differences in effects of various radiations. It is best defined by an example: If neutrons are several times more effective in causing some injury than are gamma rays of an equal energy, then that difference can be expressed as a numerical factor, which is the R.B.E. The R.B.E. for a given situation depends upon the specific physical natures of the radiations being compared and the biological effect which is being studied. The R.B.E. for neutrons when compared with gamma rays may be very high (10 to 20) when the biological end point is cataract formation, whereas it may be quite modest (1.0 to 3.0) when mortality rates are being measured. The overall or net R.B.E. for neutrons from weapons has been accepted as 1.0.

d. Rem. An abbreviation for the term "Roentgen Equivalent Man (or Mammal)." This term describes irradiation as a biological dose. It was designed to be related to the clinical effect seen and, therefore, to be independent of the form of irradiation. It has an obvious disadvantage in that it cannot be directly measured, but must be calculated. The rad has become a preferred term for most usage.

e. Radioactive Half-Life. The time required for the activity of a given radioactive isotope to decrease to half its initial value due to radioactive decay. The half-life is a characteristic property of each radioactive isotope and is independent of its amount or condition.

f. Biological Half-Time. The time required for the amount of a specified element which has entered the body (or a particular organ) to be decreased to half its initial value as a result of natural, biological elimination processes.

g. Effective Half-Life. The time in which the quantity of a given isotope in the body will decrease to half as a result of radioactive decay and biological elimination.

17. Nuclear Radiation Injury

a. Cellular Sensitivity. All tissues and cells are not equally sensitive to radiation injury. Certain tissues and cells, including the lymphoid tissue, the hematopoietic part of the bone marrow, and mature lymphocytes, are especially sensitive. Accordingly, at moderate doses, injury to these tissues, with resultant under-production or over-production of metabolic products, hormones, specialized cells, and enzymes, alteration of growth rates of all populations, or death of cells and tissues, determines the type of clinical response. Other tissues, the mucosa of the gastrointestinal tract for example, are moderately sensitive to radiation injury. However, gut damage becomes clinically obvious sooner than does bone marrow damage. Therefore, with higher doses, injury to the gut determines the clinical picture. Resistant or relatively resistant cells and tissues include nerve cells, bone, and the eyes. With large prompt doses, the clinical result of injury to these structures becomes manifest before the injuries to the more sensitive parts have time to become manifest. Why cells or tissues which require higher doses to show clinical defects do so sooner is not known but has been related to different mechanisms of damage. The bone marrow and gut effects are probably due to effects on cell regeneration patterns, whereas the CNS effects are probably due to alterations of cell function and associated cell injury or death. Table 8 shows the relative sensitivities of a large number of mammalian cells. Cells in the same category have roughly the same sensitivity.

b. The Syndrome of Radiation Sickness and Factors Which Vary It. Radiation injury to man results in a variety of clinical patterns depending upon the interaction of several variables. These variables must be considered when radiation injury is classified and described. They include the amount of body exposed, the physical nature of the radiation, the total dose received, the dose rate

Table 8. Categories of Mammalian Cell Sensitivities (Based on Morphologic Criteria of Cell Death) Progression From Most to Least Sensitive Groupings

I.	Lymphocytes, especially small lymphocytes Erythroblasts Spermatogonia B
II.	Granulosa cells in developing and mature ovarian follicles Myelocytes Intestinal crypt cells Germinal cells of epidermis
III.	Gastric gland cells Endothelial cells small blood vessels
IV.	Osteoblasts Osteoclasts Chondroblasts Granulosa cells primitive ovarian follicles Spermatocytes Spermatids
V.	Granulocytes and thrombocytes Osteocytes Spermatozoa Superficial cells of GI tract
VI.	Parenchymal and duct cells of glands Fibroblasts Endothelial cells of large blood vessels Erythrocytes
VII.	Fibrocytes Reticular cells Chondrocytes Phagocytes
VIII.	Muscle cells Nerve cells

and number of exposures, and the physiological state of the exposed man.

(1) *Whole-body vs partial-body irradiation.* The proportion of the body which is exposed to radiation is a major factor in determining the nature and degree of morbidity and the probability of mortality.

(a) The most serious clinical disturbances and highest probability of death follow whole-body irradiation. This can occur as a result or exposure to the gamma rays and neutrons emitted at the instant of detonation of a weapon or the gamma rays in a fallout field, or by the internal deposition of such isotopes as tritium, cesium–137, and carbon–14 which distribute themselves uniformly throughout the body.

(b) Partial-body irradiation will cause a variety of clinical effects, depending upon the ratio of exposed to unexposed tissue and the sparing or nonsparing of critical tissue. The less tissue exposed, the less severe will be the morbidity, the less likely will be mortality, and the higher will be the dose per gram of tissue iradiated which can be tolerated. When soldiers are exposed to prompt or initial radiation from a weapon or to fallout, their positions relative to the environment may result in significant shielding of parts of their bodies. Soldiers in foxholes, in vehicles, and in buildings will all be shielded to some extent. The most critical tissue to be shielded is the bone marrow, and a soldier subjected to half-body irradiation, lower or upper, could have significant sparing of his bone marrow. If the total dose of irradiation received is not in the very high or supralethal range, such a soldier could develop significant symptoms and signs of radiation injury, yet survive. His clinical condition during much of this illness could not be distinguished easily from whole-body irradiation with a much higher probability of mortality (close to 100 percent). This is discussed further in paragraph 18. Concentration of isotopes within certain organs can occur. Iodine in the thyroid and strontium in the bone are examples. Significant damage can occur to specific tissue as a result, and long term effects can follow. This is a long term hazard of fallout, and is discussed further in paragraph 22.

(2) *Physical nature of radiation.* The physical nature of the radiation will determine the pattern of injury to tissue.

(*a*) Gamma or X-radiations are the most penetrating and can cause damage throughout the full thickness of a human body. The degree of penetration is energy-dependent in that very low energy or "soft" X-rays do not penetrate deeply into tissue, whereas high energy "X" or gamma rays will. The gamma radiation associated with nuclear weapons is generally energetic enough to be deeply penetrating.

(*b*) Neutrons are less penetrating than are gamma rays of equivalent energy. Since they are absorbed more rapidly, they lose more energy in a given depth of tissue and cause more damage in the superficial layers of the tissue. This phenomenon is energy dependent, and very high energy neutrons can penetrate through the whole body thickness. However, since the neutrons emitted by the fission process of a nuclear weapon cover a wide range of energies, more damage will occur in the superficial tissue on the side facing the detonation.

(*c*) Neutrons and gamma rays are emitted together from a weapon. As a result, the biological effects would be mixed. The net clinical effects would in general reflect the injury due to the more penetrating gamma radiation which is more apt to be whole body in its distribution of energy deposition. An exception to this could occur when shielding prevents whole-body exposure. Certain superficial areas are particularly sensitive to neutron irradiation. These are the lens of the eye, discussed in paragraphs 10 and 20, and those areas of the skin which are over bony prominences, such as the scalp, hips, and shoulders. In these areas, severe skin damage can occur. These lesions require many weeks to develop and are discussed in paragraph 20.

(*d*) Beta particles do not penetrate deeply. Most of the fission products resulting from a nuclear detonation are beta emitters. The primary clinical hazard would be skin burns due to prolonged contact of the fission products with the skin.

(*e*) Alpha particles are heavily charged particles which do not constitute a hazard when outside the body since the most superficial part of the keratin layer of the skin will absorb them. They are a hazard when deposited and retained internally. Aerosols of plutonium as a fine dust or fume can be retained in pulmonary tissue, and the alpha radiation which would result would cause damage over a long period of time. This is also discussed in paragraph 21.

(3) *Dose of radiation.* Both the type of clinical syndrome produced and its severity are dose dependent. The typical clinical syndromes (para 18) which follow whole-body irradiation occur within characteristic dose ranges. A similar dose-dependent relationship exists for type of syndrome and its severity following partial body or localized irradiation.

(4) *Dose rate and fractionation.* The dose rate of the radiation will determine the amount of energy required to produce equal biological effects.

(*a*) As the dose rate of radiation increases, the amount of energy required to produce a given effect decreases. This is particularly true of gamma or X-irradiation, but less so of neutron-irradiation. In combat, the difference between the high dose rate of the mixed radiation emitted on detonation, and the variable but lower dose rates of the gamma component of fallout fields could be large enough for a dose rate effect to be present. However, the clinical patterns which irradiated patients would show would not give a clue as to the dose rate of the exposure. Therefore, treatment decisions would have to be based on clinical evidence regardless of what dose or dose rate caused the problem.

(*b*) Fractionation of irradiation into several separate doses will be characterized by a certain amount of recovery or repair between doses. The longer the time intervals, the more the recovery or repair. There is an irreducible minimum of injury which remains after each dose and which accumulates with each successive dose. This phenomenon has been seen experimentally with both gamma and neutron irradiation.

(5) *Physiological Factors.* The physiological state of the individual when exposed will have a variable effect upon morbidity and probability of mortality.

(a) *Age.* Both the very young and the very old are more sensitive than are young healthy adults.

(b) *Physiologic changes with stress.* Evidence suggests that moderate to severe physical stress, prior to irradiation, which is well tolerated, may increase resistance to radiation injury. Poorly tolerated or post-irradiation stresses both tend to increase the severity of the response to radiation injury. The timing of the stress in relation to radiation exposure and the degree of the stress are both highly critical. The pituitary-adrenal axis has been incriminated in these phenomena, but the exact nature of its role is not clear. In combat with its multiple stresses, the result would be increased variability of response in a given population to given radiation doses.

(c) *Concurrent or pre-existent disease.* The interactions of radiation with concurrent or pre-existent disease is largely unknown, although it is reasonable to expect that the addition of radiation injury to the burden of pre-existing disease would be deleterious. There is evidence that whole-body irradiation may uncover latent or subclinical infections. In addition, it has been suggested that irradiation at the time of immunization with live organisms will result in generalized disease. This last finding has not been fully investigated, and specific recommendations as to changes in the immunization schedules now in effect cannot be given at this time.

18. The Acute Radiation Syndrome and its Management

a. *General*

(1) The prognosis and treatment of radiation injury depend upon the clinical picture presented by the patient. The clinical pictures or syndromes are related to the dose of irradiation sustained, although the dose-effect relationship will be modified by the variables described in paragraph 17. This variability makes dosimetry data of little use when diagnostic or treatment decisions must be made on individual patients.

(2) The syndromes to be described in the following paragraphs are characteristic of whole-body irradiation, although partial-body irradiation can often result in similar clinical patterns. Also discussed are a number of clinical problems which would result from high dose partial-body or localized irradiation.

(3) Three syndromes, commonly termed the Central-Nervous, Gastrointestinal, and Hematopoietic Syndromes, form a well recognized group, classified according to the organ system which is responsible for the predominant signs and symptoms. These syndromes form a spectrum of clinical response which is dose-dependent. They have three characteristic survival times which are shown graphically in figure 7.

(4) It will be noted that the limit of 100 percent probability of mortality is rather low on the scale, somewhere between the hematopoietic and gastrointestinal parts of the curve. This is characteristic of whole-body irradiation.

b. *Central Nervous System Syndrome.*

(1) Very high (supralethal) whole-body doses will result in a clinical course reflecting severe effects upon the central nervous system. The minimum dose required (for single, acute, high dose rate exposures) is estimated at about 3,000 to 5,000 rads for man. The dosage above which death essentially becomes instantaneous and is no longer due to CNS effects is unknown for man, but is speculated to be in the region of 50,000 rads or greater.

(2) In combat, it is unlikely that individuals subjected to extremely high doses (50,000 rads and above) would survive to be seen in medical facilities, but survivors of exposures in the range of 3,000 to 10,000 rads may reach forward medical units. Weapons, 2 KT and above, have such large blast and thermal yields that no individuals close enough to receive such high doses of irradiation would survive. Smaller weapons present relatively greater radiation hazards, and it is possible for individuals who are protected from blast and thermal effects, to receive high enough doses of radiation to develop the CNS syndrome.

(3) The pathophysiology of this syndrome is not known. The pathological findings are mild and do not provide substantial clues. Typically, small, fairly localized, perivascular hemorrhages and moderate edema are present. Neuronal changes have been described, but are not constant. Localized irradiation of the head alone will result in a similar clinical picture and similar pathological findings, but only with doses of much greater magnitudes.

(4) Typically, victims with this syndrome have an early transient phase of incapacitation with marked ataxia lasting a few minutes to less than an hour. This would rarely be seen by a military physician in combat situations. It is followed by a variable period of lucidity. Sometime during the next 2 hours to 3 days, a severe, rapid, clinical deterioration would begin with alternating pe-

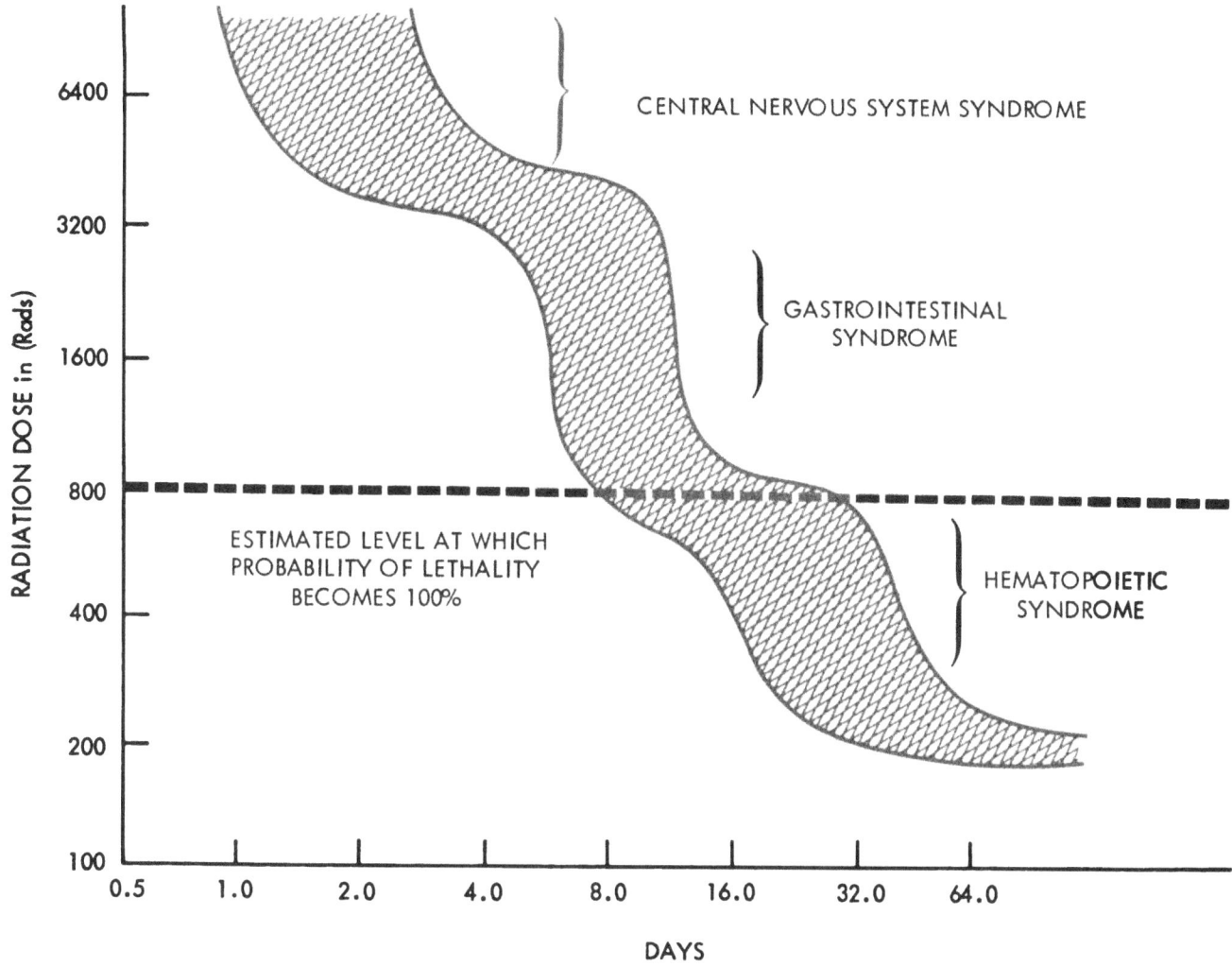

Figure 7. Survival times in days.

riods of lethargy and hyperactivity, and with grand-mal convulsions and ataxia. This would be followed by a period of deepening come culminating in cardiovascular collapse and death. The total period of time involved is highly variable, from as short as a few hours to as long as 3 days.

(5) The typical patient would not be seen in a medical facility until after the onset of the second phase of more severe incapacitation. He would present as a patient with serious CNS disease, without localizing signs or clinical signs of severe cerebral edema. Examination of cerebrospinal fluid would not reveal abnormalities. There is no specific test available at this time which would allow the diagnosis of radiation injury of the CNS to be made. With the high doses involved, neutron-induced radioactivity would be present in tissues and body fluids. No practical field test has yet been standardized which would take advantage of this phenomenon.

(6) Victims of accidental exposures to high doses have shown a marked flushing of the skin which may wax and wane. The mechanism for this is not understood and too few cases have occurred to establish whether this is a pathognomonic sign of severe radiation injury.

(7) The mortality in patients with the CNS syndrome, is 100 percent regardless of treatment, and only supportive and symptomatic treatment is indicated. When the situation requires sorting for treatment or movement, these patients should be given a low priority.

c. Gastrointestinal Syndrome.

(1) Radiation doses in the range of 750 rads to 3,000 rads will result in a characteristic syndrome of bloody diarrhea, fever, and dehydration. The pathological changes underlying this clinical picture include inflammatory and necrotic changes in the gastrointestinal tract, seen during the first week after exposure.

(2) During the first few hours after irradiation, there may be a short period of time during which nausea, vomiting, and malaise may occur. This may be followed by a period of relative well-

being. The actual symptomatic phase of the gastrointestinal syndrome would begin between the third to seventh day. This is the time when the denudation of the gastrointestinal mucosa would result in fluid losses and hemorrhage severe enough to incapacitate the individual.

(3) With a reliable history of exposure and the knowledge that the patient does not have significant gastrointestinal disease on some other basis, the diagnosis poses no problem. Also, if the patient's peripheral blood count presents a typical severe lymphopenia with a moderate to marked leukopenia, the presumptive diagnosis of radiation injury could be made. Differential diagnosis may be difficult when the history of exposure is in doubt and/or the peripheral blood counts do not show marked depressions. Partial-body irradiation, particularly with exposure of the gut, can give a picture similar to that given by whole-body irradiation. Diarrheal disease due to infection, may likewise be present at the same time as effects of small, less serious doses of irradiation. Positive stool cultures or smears may give a clue, but these do not rule out severe radiation injury.

(4) The diagnosis of radiation injury cannot be firmly established under these circumstances. Patients who have the gastrointestinal syndrome due to whole-body irradiation have little chance for survival. Those who have had partial-body exposure may recover, although the prognosis is guarded. Those who have a combination of diseases, wherein an infectious disease is responsible for the gastrointestinal problems and this is complicated by mild radiation injury, may also have a chance for recovery. The inability to differentiate easily among these different conditions requires the responsible medical officer to be cautious about deciding prematurely that a particular patient's condition is hopeless.

(5) Treatment of patients with the gastrointestinal syndrome is symptomatic and supportive with heavy reliance on fluids and electrolytes. If the patient can be sustained through the first few days, he will then enter a period of bone marrow depression with its attendant syndrome of hemorrhage and susceptibility to infection discussed below. The probability of lethality remains very high under the most favorable circumstances since the degree of bone marrow depression will be severe. Patients with even partial protection of their bone marrow by shielding would have a very much better chance of survival because the depression of bone marrow activity would be less likely to be to dangerous levels.

d. *Hematopoietic Snydrome.*

(1) This syndrome occurs when patients receive doses of irradiation too low to cause the gastrointestinal syndrome, or when patients are in the latter phase of a mild gastrointestinal syndrome (table 9). It is the most important clinical problem to be faced because it is seen over a wide range of doses both lethal and sublethal. Patients with even very low levels of whole-body irradiation with a high probability of survival will still show some degree of bone marrow depression. Therefore, when a patient is seen with bone marrow depression due to irradiation, in the absence of the GI or CNS syndrome, it should be assumed that the injury is sublethal, unless it is *known* to be otherwise.

(2) The hematopoietic syndrome may be divided into the following phases: Exposure phase, delay time, initial (or prodromal) phase, latent phase, secondary phase of overt hypoplastic anemia, and convalescence phase.

(*a*) The exposure phase is the time during which the radiation is received, while the delay time refers to the period from time of exposure to the onset of initial symptoms of the initial or prodromal reaction. This delay time lasts a few hours.

(*b*) The initial or prodromal phase is characterized by a prodromal reaction (nausea, vomiting, and fatigue), usually lasting 2 to 3 days. This reaction may be very mild and may not even occur.

(*c*) The period from the subsidence of the initial or prodromal symptoms, if they occur, to the onset of overt hypoplastic anemia is called the latent phase and is usually about 3 weeks long. It is most probable that casualties will not become patients until they are past the latent phase.

(*d*) The secondary phase of overt hypoplastic anemia occurs 3 to 6 weeks following radiation exposure. Epilation, which usually occurs about 2 weeks following exposure to 300 rads or more, will frequently herald the onset of this phase of the injury and may be a significant clinical sign. If it does occur, then the victim is likely to develop a significant hematopoietic syndrome.

(*e*) The convalescent phase begins approximately 3 months post-exposure. By this time, hematopoietic recovery will usually have progressed to such a point that the threat of complications has subsided, and the patient would no longer need hospitalization or frequent medical observation.

(3) The most important phase clinically is that of the overt hypoplastic anemia. The basic problems which are seen during this phase are hemorrhage and susceptibility to infection.

(*a*) The hemorrhagic manifestations are due to the thrombocytopenia. When platelet depression reaches a critical level, mucosal bleeding

Table 9. Acute Clinical Effects of Single High Dose Rate Exposures of Whole-Body Irradiation to Healthy Adults

Dose (Range)	0-100 rads (subclinical range)	100-1000 rads (sublethal range)			Over 1000 rads (lethal range)	
		100-200 rads	200-600 rads	600-1000 rads	1000-3000 rads	over 3000 rads
INITIAL PHASE — Incidence of nausea & vomiting	NONE	5-50%	50-100%	75-100%	100%	
Time of onset		Approx. 3-6 hrs.	Approx. 2-4 hrs.	Approx 1-2 hrs.	Less than 1 hr	
Duration		Less than 24 hrs.	Less than 24 hrs.	Less than 48 hrs.	Less than 48 hrs.	Approx 48 hrs.
Combat effectiveness	100%	100%	Can perform routine tasks. Sustained combat or comparable activities hampered for 6-20 hrs.	Can perform only simple routine tasks. Significant incapacitation in upper part of range. Lasts more than 24 hrs.	Progressive incapacitation following an early capability for intermittent heroic response.	Progressive incapacitation following an early capability for intermittent heroic response.
LATENT PHASE — Duration		More than 2 weeks.	Approx. 7-15 days.	None to approx 7 days.	None to approx 2 days.	NONE
Signs & symptoms	NONE	Moderate leukopenia.	Severe leukopenia; purpura, hemorrhage; Infection; epilation about 300 rads.		Diarrhea; fever; disturbance of electrolyte balance	Convulsions; tremor; ataxia; lethargy
SECONDARY PHASE — Time of onset post exposure.		2 weeks or more.	Several days to 2 weeks		2-3 days	
Critical period post exposure.	NONE	NONE	4-6 weeks		5-14 days	1-48 hrs
Organ system responsible.	NONE	Hematopoietic tissue			Gastrointestinal tract	Central nervous system
HOSPITALIZATION — Percentage	NONE	Less than 5%	90%	100%	100%	100%
Duration		45-60 days	60-90 days	90-120 days	2 weeks	2 days
INCIDENCE OF DEATH	NONE	NONE	0-80%	90-100%	90-100%	
AVERAGE TIME OF DEATH			3 weeks to 2 months		1-2 weeks	2 days
THERAPY	NONE	Reassurance hematologic surveillance	Blood transfusion, antibiotics		Maintenance of electrolyte balance.	Sedatives

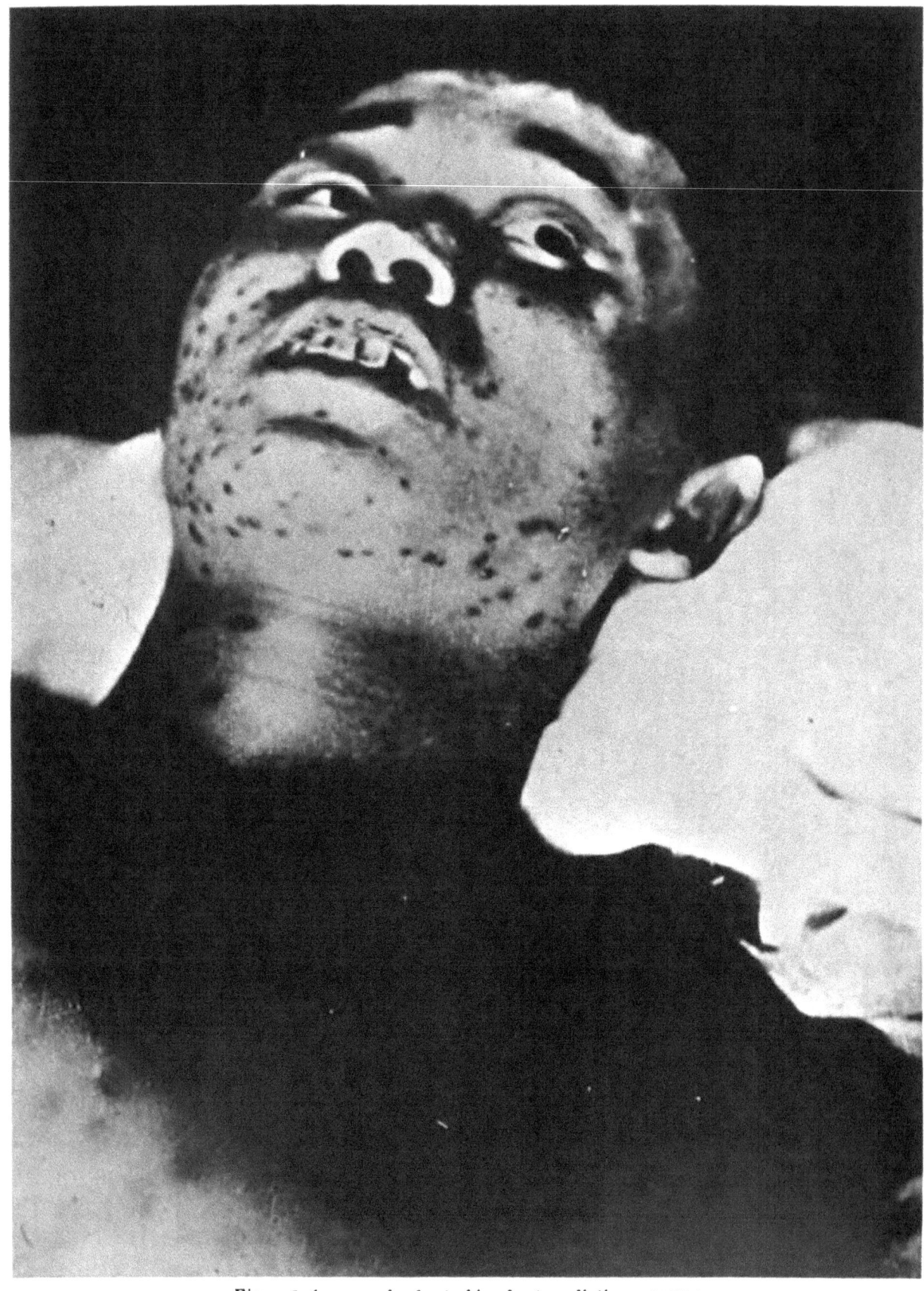

Figure 8. An example of petechiae due to radiation exposure.

28

becomes common. The first signs will be epistaxis and gingival bleeding. Later, gastrointestinal and pulmonary bleeding will occur in the more heavily exposed patients. Coagulation times will be prolonged and multiple subcutaneous petechiae will be common (fig. 8). Ideally, treatment should include platelet transfusions. An acceptable alternative is fresh whole blood. If neither is available, the prognosis is guarded.

(b) The second threat to life is infection. This is complicated by a depression of the normal physiological response to infection. A patient may develop an overwhelming sepsis without the characteristic signs and symptoms. The liberal use of antibiotics is indicated. Bactericidal drugs are preferred over bacterostatic.

(4) The effect of irradiation in this dose range on latent and subclinical infections and on carrier states is unknown. Research evidence to date, though, would support the hypothesis that the results of irradiation in such circumstances would be deleterious. Also, organisms which would normally not be pathogens might cause significant morbidity and mortality. This would apply even to immunizations with live organisms. Research has suggested that the combination of whole-body irradiation and immunization with live organisms may result in generalized, fatal, infectious disease. However, until positive evidence has substantiated this further, the present immunization programs should be continued in nuclear warfare.

e. *Diagnostic Clues.* Evaluation of the following findings, if early medical evaluation of victims is possible, will be helpful in estimating the severity of nuclear radiation injury:

(1) *Clinical diagnosis.*

(a) *Nausea and vomiting.* Although of little prognostic value for the individual person, these initial or prodromal symptoms could be of some prognostic significance for large groups of casualties. The absence of these symptoms within 4 hours post-exposure indicates that exposure has been limited to insignificant amounts of irradiation and that the need for hospitalization will not arise. On the other hand, when an appreciable percentage of a group exhibits vomiting within 2 hours, exposures to significant amounts of irradiation have probably occurred, and incapacitation requiring hospitalization of some individuals can be anticipated.

(b) *Latent phase.* The duration of the latent phase is also of some prognostic value. With the onset of hemorrhage or infection after a 3-week latent period, the typical hematopoietic form of the illness may be anticipated. However, when a clear latent period is not evident or when its duration is much shorter than 3 weeks, the prognosis is more serious. *For example,* the development of symptoms (diarrhea, severe vomiting and abdominal pain) within a few days post-exposure may herald the onset of the gastrointestinal form of the illness.

(c) *Fever.* In the hematopoietic form of the injury, fever may be seen at the end of the third week, but it does not necessarily indicate a poor prognosis. However, high fever occurring with a few days following exposure may indicate the onset of the gastrointestinal syndrome and thus a high probability of mortality.

(d) *Epilation.* Loss of hair about 2 weeks after irradiation indicates a significant exposure to 300 rads or more (fig. 9). All patients with excessive loss of hair should be observed closely because this finding usually occurs about 1 week prior to signs of hematopoietic injury, and thus indicates the need for future observation and treatment. If possible, such patients should be hospitalized because, even though they appear well, they would soon enter a period of severely increased susceptibility to a variety of complications, particularly infection. However, other considerations could preclude this plan of management, and no rigid theater medical policy could be established.

(e) *Diarrhea.* Early, persistent diarrhea is a serious prognostic sign and indicates exposure to more than 400 rads and the existence of significant gastrointestinal damage as discussed above.

(2) *Laboratory Diagnosis.*

(a) *Leukopenia.* The total white blood cell count is likely to be at the lowest point between the fourt and sixth weeks following exposure. Clinical illness is unlikely if the total white blood count remains about 2,500. However, when the count ranges between 1,000 and 2,500, the typical hematopoietic form of the injury will be manifested; and patients with counts below 1,000 will usually have a serious clinical course.

(b) *Lymphopenia.* In contrast to the polymorphonuclear leucocyte count, lymphopenia may be noted within 48 hours following exposure. The lymphocyte count during this period is of limited value in estimating the severity of injury since it is depressed profoundly by such low doses of irradiation. This is shown in table 10.

(c) A mild, transient leukocytosis can occur prior to the severe leukopenia. Therefore, normal to elevated white counts during the latent phase after known exposures cannot be considered a good prognostic sign.

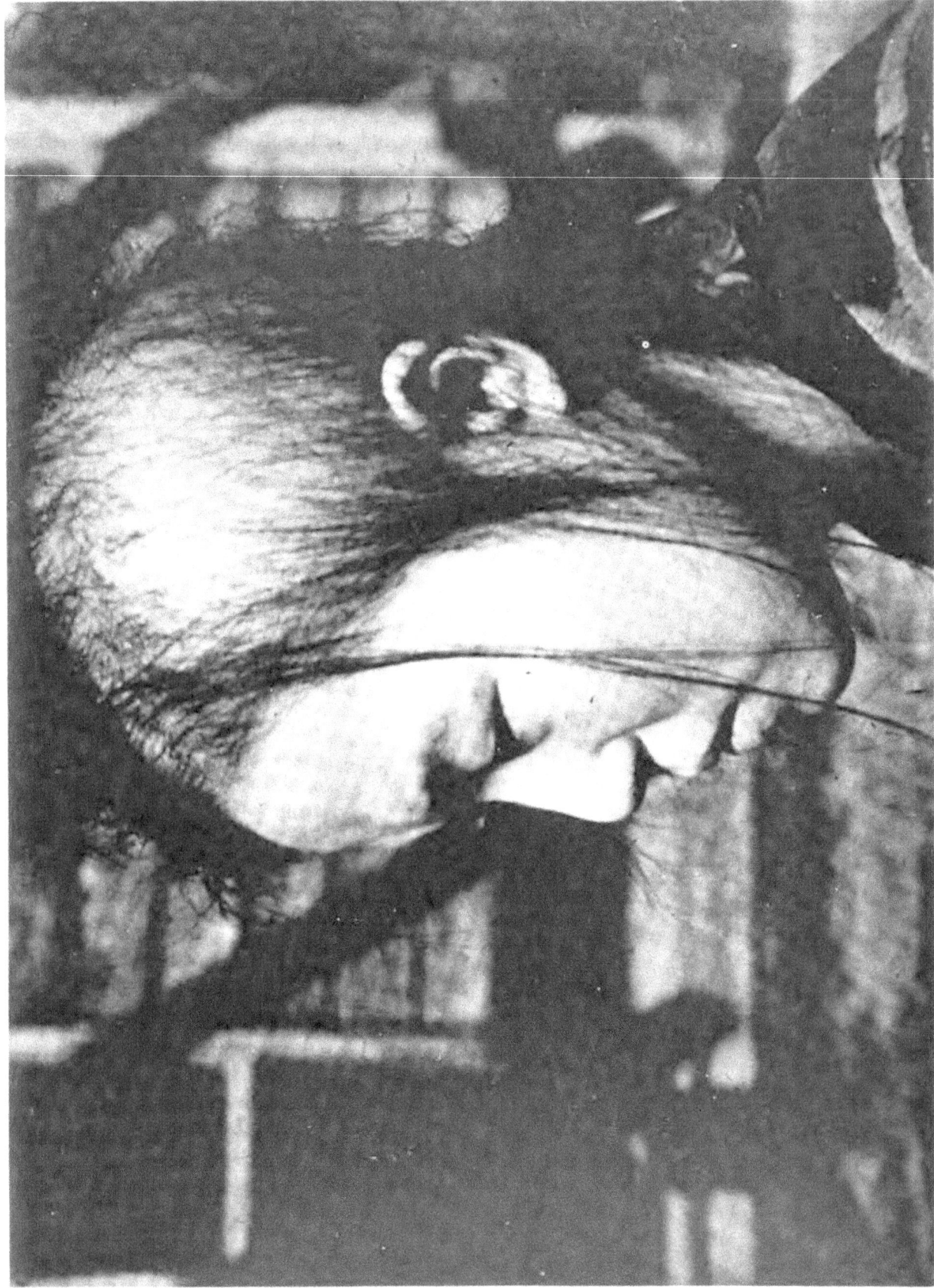

Figure 9. An example of epilation due to radiation exposure.

Table 10. *Lymphocyte Count Following Exposure*

Blood count findings	Dose
No significant decrease in count....	Less than 50 rads
Mild decrease	Less than 100 rads
More than 50 percent decrease.....	More than 100 rads

19. Combined Injury

a. After the atomic bombs were dropped in Japan, many of the patients with other injuries developed clinical signs and symptoms of radiation sickness from 1 to 3 weeks after exposure, depending on the dose received. Clinically, the gastrointestinal and hematopoietic syndromes were superimposed upon or combined with other injuries. These injuries included burns, lacerations from secondary missiles, fractures, trauma from falling debris, and internal injuries from primary blast effects. Mortality in the cases with multiple injuries which included significant signs of radiation sickness was high due to the occurrence of systemic bacterial infections, severe fluid and electrolyte losses, and the development of hemorrhagic diatheses.

b. The approach to a combined injury should include an initial survey to determine the relative contributions of each type of injury to the patient's clinical condition. Generally, each should be treated individually as outlined in other sections of this handbook. However, there are certain characteristics of combined injury which are important.

(1) The prognosis in general depends upon the severity of the wound or burn. Minor injuries which are closed such as sprains, strains and simple fractures, or simple lacerations have little effect on mortality. Large open wounds particularly burns of 20 percent or more of the body surface are very hazardous. This is reasonable since such injuries will still be "open" and potential sites of bacterial invasion during the period of bone marrow depression when resistance to infection is lowest. Therefore, management of open wounds should be directed toward the prevention and treatment of infectious complications.

(2) The timing of the injury relative to the exposure to irradiation will greatly affect the eventual outcome. Mechanical injuries which are sustained during a period of a few days prior to whole-body irradiation may actually produce an increased resistance to the irradiation and a decreased probability of mortality. Injuries sustained after irradiation, particularly from 2 to 10 days later result in markedly increased mortality. Burns sustained at almost any time prior to, during, or after whole-body irradiation may produce increased mortality. This results from the fact that the condition of the patient relative to his mechanical or thermal injury at the time of radiation exposure may not be as important as his condition at the time 3 weeks later when his bone marrow depression becomes severe.

(3) Patients who require surgery in the immediate post-irradiation period will tolerate it reasonably well if the procedure is simple and closed. If extensive debridement of extremity injuries is done with the required delayed closure of large areas, then there is an increased risk of infectious complications which will occur during the period of bone marrow depression. The other complication affecting combined injury is the hemorrhagic tendency which occurs due to bone marrow depression. This is seen from about 2 to 3 weeks after irradiation. Patients who require surgical treatment at this time will have much higher complication and mortality rates. If fresh whole blood is available, it should be used on such patients.

(4) Although simple fractures will not have a marked effect on mortality when sustained at the time of radiation exposure, the radiation will result in delayed healing. Immobilization will have to be prolonged, but this is not a problem as long as adequate X-ray facilities are available to aid in following these patients. Open fractures present the same problem of possible infectious complications as do other open wounds.

(5) Open wounds will show a transient delay in healing during the period of bone marrow depression, which occurs about 2 to 3 weeks after exposure. If the depression is not severe and recovery occurs, the wounds will then resume healing. During this time of delayed healing, the patients are very susceptible to infectious complications and may also show severe bleeding tendencies.

(6) Whole-body irradiation is associated with increased sensitivity to anesthetic agents generally. However, not enough is known about the response of man to these agents following irradiation to allow specific recommendations to be made as to the choice of agents or as to dose reduction factors. The response of the individual patient to given doses must be carefully watched.

c. The following principles should be followed in the general management of patients who may have combined injury:

(1) In order to make the diagnosis, all patients must be continuously watched for signs of whole-body irradiation such as epilation or anemia.

(2) When bone marrow depression is found in a patient the two problems of hemorrhage and infection must be watched for and treated.

(a) Adequate treatment of the hemorrhagic diathesis in the field will be difficult.

(b) Prevention and treatment of the infectious complications include—

1. Minimal handling and dressing changes of wounds if they are dry.

2. Copious irrigation and frequent wet dressings if there is infection.

3. Use of isolation techniques if the facilities are adequate and the patient load allows it.

4. The liberal use of antibiotics.

20. Cutaneous Effects of Irradiation

Cutaneous effects of clinical significance require fairly high doses of irradiation. Therefore, in whole-body irradiation which is nearly uniform, cutaneous effects are minor and are usually limited to transient erythema seen at various times following exposure. When the whole body dose is not uniform or when there is significant shielding to allow higher doses to the skin, cutaneous changes may become quite significant and disabling. Patients in this latter category have occurred as a result of accidents involving nuclear materials in industrial situations.

a. If some superficial area of the body is subjected to a considerably higher dose of irradiation than is the whole body, a pattern somewhat resembling severe second degree burns or severe cold injury will ensue.

(1) Within a short time after exposure, erythema and burning sensations will be common. These will be followed by severe, tense swelling. Blisters ensue; and, under the blisters, after several days, a dry necrosis begins.

(2) This combination of epidermolysis and dry gangrene is severely incapacitating if critical areas such as the hands or feet are involved. Also, patients who present with these types of cutaneous changes may well have sustained fatal levels of whole-body irradiation. However, if blood counts indicate the bone marrow is uninvolved, or only mildly depressed they have a good chance for survival. The skin lesions should be managed as burns.

b. If the radiation to which the skin has been exposed contains neutrons, a severe long term effect may be seen.

(1) Several weeks following exposure, ulcerations appear and gradually enlarge resembling ischemic bed sores. They extend to and may actually involve underlying muscle. They do not heal, and extensive plastic surgery would be required to repair them.

(2) The skin which overlies bony prominences, including the scalp and the skin of the shoulders, the hips, and portions of the extremities, is most sensitive to these long term ischemic effects of irradiation.

(3) These lesions should be uncommon in combat except among otherwise shielded troops who sustain heavy neutron exposures to extremities. These could be aggravated by certain conditions—

(a) Restrictive clothing.

(b) Exposure to wet cold with subsequent vascular insults due to cold injury complicating the radiation injury.

(c) Exposure to thermal injury which would also aggravate the vascular injury.

c. Beta burns result from the deposition of radioactive fallout material upon the unprotected skin. Valuable information concerning the development and healing of beta burns was obtained from observations of the Marshall Islanders who were accidentally exposed to fallout in March 1954. Some of these people allowed the fission products to remain in contact with their skin for a considerable time and the following clinical changes were seen:

(1) During the first 24 to 48 hours, a number of individuals in the highly contaminated groups experienced itching and a burning sensation of the skin. With a day or two, these early skin symptoms subsided; but, after a lapse of 2 to 3 weeks, epilation and more severe skin lesions began to develop.

(2) The first evidence of skin damage was increased pigmentation in the form of dark colored patches and raised areas. These superficial lesions developed on the exposed parts of the body not protected by clothing. Blistering was uncommon. After the formation of dry scabs, the lesions healed rapidly.

(3) Individuals who had been more highly contaminated developed deeper lesions, usually on the feet or neck. These lesions were wet, weeping, and ulcerated (fig. 10). They were painful, and many patients also complained of itching and burning. However, the majority healed readily with simple treatment.

(4) Individuals, who bathed during their exposures and who washed off the beta contamination, did not develop skin lesions. Therefore, if beta emitting contamination from fallout is removed from the skin, clinical injury should be prevented.

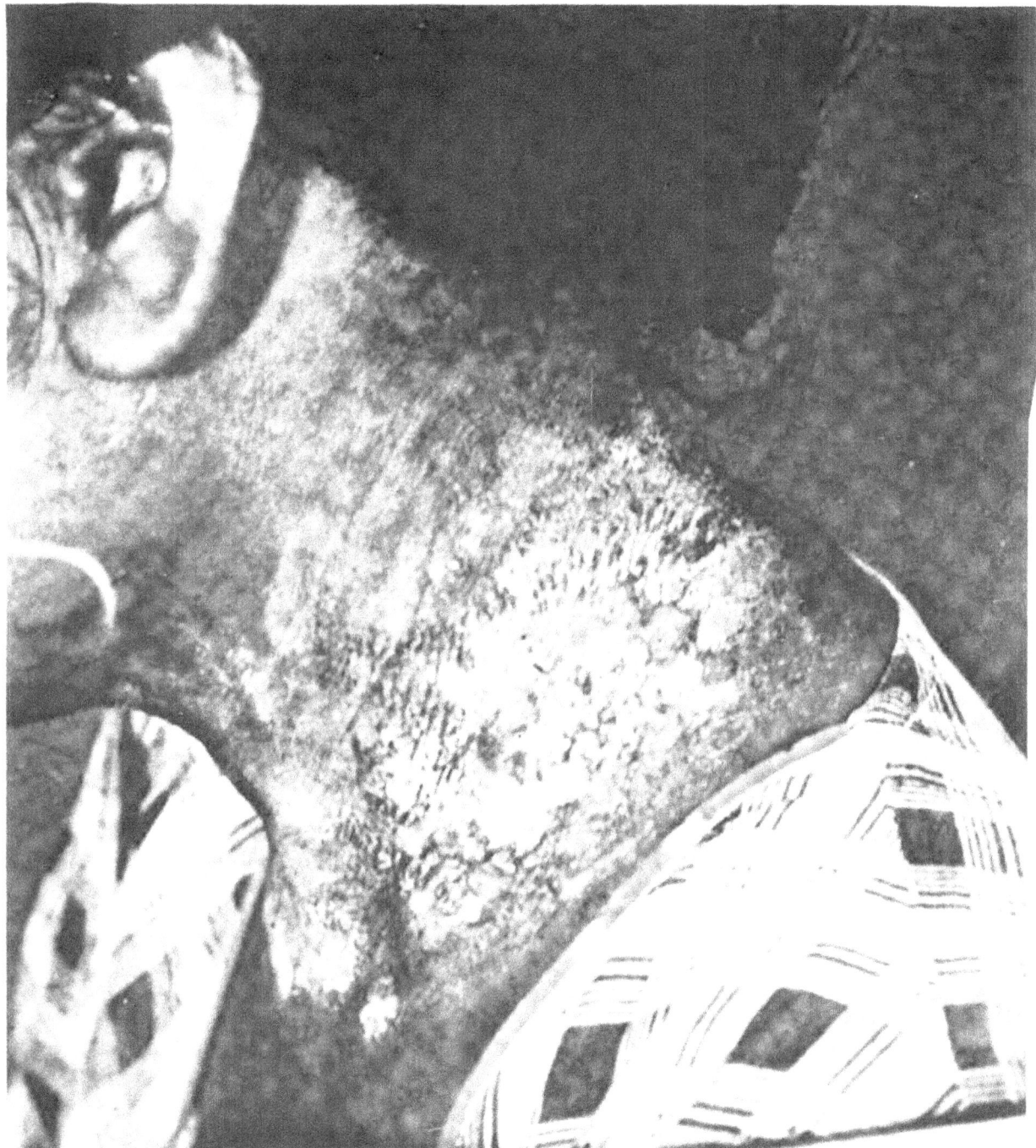

Figure 10. An example of beta burns. Neck lesions at 28 days after exposure.

(5) The acute dose-effect relationship from beta radiation absorbed in the skin is shown in table 11.

21. Effects of Internal Emitters

a. Exposure to fallout results in the hazard of radioactive materials being taken into the body through ingestion, inhalation, or absorption through wounds. Such materials inside the body are referred to as internal emitters. Radiation exposure of various organs and tissues from these internal emitters is continuous, modified only by radioactive decay and biological elimination. Internal emitters in general dissipate a significant amount of energy within a small volume of surrounding body tissue. Very low energy radiations can, therefore, cause severe tissue damage; and, if the particular element is diffusely enough distributed, severe, generalized irradiation damage can occur.

b. The fate and distribution of internal emitters are determined by the chemical nature of the

Table 11. Acute Effects From Beta Radiation Absorbed in the Skin.

Beta radiation dose (rads)	Effect
0– 600	No acute effect.
600– 2,000	Moderate early erythema.
2,000– 4,000	Early erythema under 24 hours. Skin breakdown in 2 weeks.
4,000– 10,000	Severe erythema in less than 24 hours.
10,000– 15,000	Severe erythema in less than 4 hours. Skin breakdown in 1–2 weeks.
15,000–100,000	Immediate skin blistering (less than 1 day).

elements and compounds involved. A radioisotope of an element which is a normal constituent of the body will have the same distribution and pathways as the naturally occurring, nonradioactive isotope. An example is radioactive iodine which is concentrated in the thyroid gland and incorporated into the thyroid hormone. An element not usually found in the body is usually distributed and metabolized in a manner similar to that of a normally present and chemically similar element. Thus the fission products, strontium and barium, which are similar chemically to calcium, will become incorporated into the crystals of bone. The radioisotopes of the rare earth elements, e.g., cerium, which constitute a considerable proportion of the fission products, and plutonium, which may be present to some extent in the fallout, are also "bone-seekers." Since they are not chemically similar to calcium, however, the mechanism of deposit differs from that of calcium. The difference is not important clinically, since the hazard from all of these is basically the same, i.e., damage to the bone and to the bone marrow.

c. The extent to which fallout contamination enters the blood stream depends upon two main factors: 1) particle size and, 2) solubility in body fluids. Whether or not the material is subsequently concentrated in specific tissues is determined by its chemical properties. Elements which do not tend to concentrate in a particular tissue or organ of the body are eliminated fairly rapidly.

d. The amount of radioactive material absorbed from fallout by inhalation appears to be relatively small. The reason is that the nasal air passages can filter out almost all particles with diameter greater than 10 microns (0.001 centimeter), and about 95 percent of those with diameter exceeding 5 microns (.0005 centimeter). Most particles descending in fallout during the critical period of highest activity, e.g., within 24 hours of the explosion, have diameters considerably greater than 10 microns. Consequently, only a small proportion of

the early fallout particles present in the air are sufficiently small to penetrate beyond the nasopharynx. Most of those which do penetrate into the bronchopulmonary system will be deposited on the ciliated respiratory epithelium and unless rapidly absorbed will be eliminated from the lungs within a matter of hours. Only those very small particles which can penetrate to the alveolar spaces have a measurable probability of being retained. Of those which are retained, insoluble material will remain in the alveolar region, and soluble material will be absorbed quickly into the blood stream. With time, the insoluble material is absorbed and concentrated in the lymphatic system of the lungs. The material which is removed by ciliary action higher in the bronchopulmonary tree will be swallowed and pass through the gastrointestinal tract.

e. The extent of absorption of fission products and other radioactive materials from the intestine depends upon solubility and biochemical factors. In early fallout, fission products as well as uranium and plutonium are present as oxides, many of which are not readily soluble and absorbed. Strontium and barium oxides are soluble and are absorbed through the intestinal tract and deposited in bone. Iodine is also present in a soluble form, and is, therefore, absorbed and concentrated in thyroid tissue.

f. The main hazard from a given radioactive isotope inside the body is the total radiation dose delivered to tissues while it is in the body. The most important factors in determining this dose are: isotope concentration in tissue, the nature and energy of the radiations emitted, physical half-life of the radioisotope, and the length of time the isotope remains in the tissue. The last factor is dependent upon the rate of elimination of the particular isotope, ordinarily an exponential function, and is usually expressed as the "biological half-time," which was defined earlier as the time required for one-half of a particular material introduced into the body to be eliminated from it. Combination of the radioactive half-life and biological half-time gives rise to the "effective half-life." In most cases the effective half-life in the whole body is essentially the same as that in the principal tissue or organ in which the element tends to concentrate. For some isotopes, particularly heavy metals, body radioactivity cannot be expressed in terms of a single effective half-life because their elimination does not follow simple exponential curves.

g. The isotopes which produce the greatest potential internal hazard are those with relatively short radioactive half-lives and comparatively long biological half-times. A given number of atoms of an isotope with short radioactive half-life will emit radiation at a greater rate than will the same number of atoms of another isotope, even of the same element, having a longer half-life. A long biological half-time means that a radioactive material will not be rapidly eliminated from the body. *For example*, iodine has a fairly long biological half-time in many individuals. The normal value varies over a wide range, from a few days to many years, but on the average it is about 90 days. Iodine is quickly concentrated in the thyroid gland from which it is slowly released. The radioisotope iodine–131, a fairly common fission product, has a radioactive half-life of only 8 days. Therefore, for this isotope, the conditions of short radioactive half-life and long biological half-time combine to produce serious hazard to the thyroid gland, depending upon the total amount of radioactivity absorbed.

h. For a few hours after a detonation, other radioisotopes of iodine, e.g., iodine–133 and –135, are present and contribute materially to the total hazard to the thyroid gland in an individual exposed during this interval. However, radioactive half-lives of these isotopes are measured in hours, and decay to insignificant levels occurs within a few days, and these isotopes do not contribute significantly to hazard in an individual exposed to fallout a few days after a detonation.

i. In addition to radioiodine, the most important potentially hazardous fission products are strontium–90, cesium–137, and carbon–14. Strontium–90 and cesium–137 are the more important since they can be ingested with contaminated vegetables.

(1) Strontium–90, a weak beta emitter, is incorporated into the crystals of bone. High concentrations may result in bone necrosis with severe scarring, bony tumors (sarcomas), aplastic anemia, and possibly leukemia. About 90 percent of the strontium–90 is excreted during the first 2 years after absorption, with a biological half-life varying from 40–500 days. After the first 2 years, the effective biological half-life is 18 years.

(2) Cesium–137, a weak beta and gamma emitter, is distributed the same as is potassium and thus is incorporated within all cells of the body. It, therefore, will present a whole-body hazard.

(3) Although carbon–14 emits only beta radiation, it represents a whole-body hazard because of its wide distribution and potentially long retention in the body.

j. Another potentially hazardous element, which may be present to some extent in early fall-out, is the alpha emitter, plutonium 239. This isotope has a long radioactive half-life (24,000 years) as well as a long biological half-time (about 200 years). Consequently, once it is deposited in the body and incorporated into bone, the amount present and its activity decrease at very slow rates. In spite of their short range in tissue, the continued action of alpha particles over a period of years can cause significant injury. In sufficient amounts, radium, which has a hazard similar to that of plutonium, is known to cause necrosis, and tumors of the bone, and fatal anemia. Experimental evidence indicates that less than 10 percent of inhaled plutonium is retained in the lungs. The remainder is transferred rapidly by ciliary action into the nasopharynx, where it is swallowed and eliminated in the feces. Most plutonium remaining in the lung is fixed in the pulmonary tissue and pulmonary lymph nodes. Very little is absorbed into the circulation because of limited solubility. The primary hazard is, therefore, to the lungs. The most frequent pulmonary change is mild, progressive fibrosis. Neoplastic changes might occur, but less frequently than fibrosis and considerably later in time, possibly many years.

k. Early treatment of patients with large burdens of internal emitters consists of either preventing absorption or speeding the elimination of the isotopes concerned. For ingested material, the use of chelating agents, DTPA and EDTA, or precipitating agents is indicated. In addition, cathartics should be given. Wounds or lacerations contaminated with insoluble materials may be at least partially decontaminated by irrigation, but when soluble materials are involved, chelates should be used to prevent absorption. In extreme cases, debridement may be necessary to remove the contaminant. However, excessive surgical destruction of normal tissue is not warranted. Radioactive contamination of wounds will not be life threatening. After absorption, elimination of the material can be somewhat accelerated by administration of large amounts of stable isotopes or the use of chelates to prevent utilization by the body. In the case of strontium–90, some beneficial results have been attained by decalcification.

22. Late Effects of Ionizing Radiation

There are a number of consequences of nuclear radiation which may not appear for some years after exposure and, therefore, do not constitute combat medical problems. However, their importance justifies a brief discussion.

a. Cataract Formation. Examination of the survivors of the bombings of Hiroshima and

Nagasaki has revealed about 100 cases of lens opacities in persons who were within about 900 meters (0.6 mile) of ground zero at the times of the explosions. In a small number of these patients, the opacities have been serious enough to require removal. Because of the relatively high biological effectiveness of fast neutrons for the formation of lens opacities, as compared with gamma rays, it is possible that neutron radiation was responsible for the Japanese cases. Most persons in the same zone with respect to the center of the explosion, died from thermal or mechanical injuries or from radiation illness. Consequently, it is probable that most of the survivors who developed cataracts received doses of radiation in the midlethal range. This view is supported by the fact that almost all these individuals suffered complete but transient epilation and many exhibited other characteristic clinical symptoms of radiation injury.

b. *Life Shortening.* Laboratory experiments with animals indicate that shortening of the life span, apart from the specific effect of induction of leukemia and other forms of fatal malignant disease, can result from partial or whole-body exposure to radiation. Such shortening may be the result of a number of factors, including decreased immunity to infection and premature aging. The life shortening in a given animal, for a specific radiation dose, apparently depends on such factors as genetic constitution and the age and physical condition at the time of exposure. During 1960 a study was made, under the direction of the Atomic Bomb Casualty Commission, on a large group of people in Hiroshima and Nagasaki to determine if there was any evidence of increased aging among survivors of the 1945 nuclear detonations. The results indicated that there is, at present, no support for the concept of a general, nonspecific acceleration of aging, exemplified by changes in the skin and hair, as a late radiation effect.

c. *Leukemia.*

(1) It has been suggested that acute or chronic exposure to moderate doses of nuclear radiation will induce leukemia. The first definitive evidence of an increase in the incidence of leukemia among the inhabitants of Hiroshima and Nagasaki was obtained in 1947. The peak apparently occurred between 1950 and 1952 and the incidence has subsequently decreased. Chronic granulocytic leukemia showed the greatest increase.

(2) Essentially all of the cases which could be attributed to radiation because of other associated symptoms, e.g., epilation, occurred among individuals who were within 1400 meters (0.9 mile) of ground zero. In this region, the minimum radiation dose, probably received over an extensive part of the body, has been estimated to be 400 to 500 rads. There appeared to be a direct relationship between the radiation dose and the probability of leukemia developing. Also, there were indications of a trend toward onset of the disease at an earlier age than normal.

d. *Carcinogenesis.* Research was initiated in 1957 in Hiroshima, comparing the frequency of malignant neoplasms, other than leukemia, in people exposed within about a mile of ground zero in 1945 with the incidence in unexposed populations. The results suggested a two- to fourfold increase over the expected frequency for neoplastic disease in some organs (lung, stomach, breast, and ovary) in exposed persons. However, a similar study made in Nagasaki did not show the same relationship. The investigation is being continued, and future reports may shed more light on the incidence of neoplastic disease following exposure to ionizing radiation.

e. *Retarded Development of Children.* Among the mothers, who were pregnant at the time of the nuclear explosions in Japan and who received sufficiently large doses to show radiation sickness, there was a marked increase over expected in the number of stillbirths and in the mortality of newly born and infant children. A study of the surviving children made 4 or 5 years later showed a slightly increased frequency of mental retardation. Maldevelopment of the teeth, attributed in injury of the roots was also noted in many of the children. Nearly all the mothers of these children —then in utero, were so close to ground zero that they must have been exposed to at least 450 rads of nuclear radiation. A comparison was made in 1952 between exposed children, whose ages ranged from less than 1 to about 14 years at the time of the explosions, and unexposed children of the same age. It showed that the former had somewhat lower average body weights and were less advanced in stature and sexual maturity. On the other hand, no significant differences were observed in various neuromuscular coordination and muscular tests.

f. *Sterility and Fertility.* Despite the high degree of radiosensitivity of some stages in the germ cell lines, this function of testes and ovaries is affected only transiently by sublethal levels of whole body irradiation with excellent recovery of normal function the usual end result. The typical response in male animals, studied in the laboratory and in a few accident cases involving man, following even low doses of whole-body or localized gonadal irradiation is an abrupt fall in the sperm count. The degree of fall is dose dependent, and azoospermia may be seen with low doses. The sterility may last several months to a few years, but general recovery does occur and normal fertility and offspring should occur. The dose required to cause similar transient sterility in the human female is not known, but is probably higher than that for man. Because of the cyclic nature of spermatogenesis, continuous doses of irradiation over long periods of time or fractionated doses are more likely to cause permanent sterility based upon animal experiments. The doses required would still be high.

g. Genetic Effects. Radiation can result in genetic effects and laboratory studies have shown increased mutation rates with small doses of irradiation. With increasing doses there is an increasing rate of mutations. Higher dose rates are more effective rad-for-rad in producing increased rates of mutations. However, mutations are still extremely infrequent and in an exposed human population the increased frequency could not be detected in subsequent generations, particularly, since many of the mutations thus induced would be lethal and thus completely self-limiting. No evidence of genetic effects in man has yet been found.

23. Radiation Effects on Medical Materiel

Since the effects of ionizing radiation on materiel are somewhat more insidious than are the well known effects of thermal radiation and blast, medical personnel should be aware of the possible types of damage which can occur as a result of exposure of materiel, particularly medicines and rations.

a. The radioactivity induced in rations will not be of major significance on the nuclear battlefield. Rations, suspected or known to contain induced activity, should be regarded as edible after about 1 week has elapsed. This time is required for normal radioactive decay processes to reduce the level of induced activity. If no other food is available, the ration will have to be eaten before 1 week after exposure, and the relatively small hazard associated will have to be accepted.

b. Certain drugs exposed to nuclear radiation may become either radioactive or lose potency. Drugs composed of such elements as sodium, calcium, phosphorus, tin, zinc, iron, chlorine, and sulfur readily become activated and may require from 2 to 5 days to permit the radioactive decay processes to reduce the level of activity. Such drugs as vitamin B_{12} and insulin are particularly prone to loss of potency and, in tests, have shown

losses of 50 percent and 10 percent of their potency respectively. As in the case of radiation activated food, the urgency of the situation, when weighed against availability of supplies, would determine whether exposed drugs would be used.

24. Protective Measures

a. Initial Nuclear Radiation. The amount of initial gamma and neutron radiation received by personnel is influenced primarily by two factors —distance and shielding.

(1) The intensity of the initial nuclear radiation decreases rapidly with distance from the point of burst due to the spread of the radiation over larger and larger areas as it travels away from the explosion and to the absorption, scattering and capture (neutrons) by the atmosphere. To illustrate, the approximate slant distances at which 100 rads, 500 rads and 1,000 rads will travel for weapons of different energy yields are shown in table 12.

Table 12. Ranges from Ground Zero for Various Initial Nuclear Radiation Doses From Airbursts

	Explosion yield				
	1 KT	10 KT	100 KT	1 MT	10 MT
Radiation dose:					
100 rads	1,100	1,600	2,100	2,900	3,900
500 rads	1,000	1,300	1,800	2,400	3,400
1,000 rads	800	1,100	1,600	2,300	3,200

It should be noted that a distance of 300 meters (low yield weapon—1 KT) to 700 meters (high yield weapon—10 MT) decreases the radiation by a factor of 10. Note also at the 1,000 rads level, a 10,000 fold increase in yield, extends the range only by a factor of 4 (800 to 3,200 meters). By dispersing troops, the effects of initial nuclear radiation can be significantly reduced.

(2) Shielding can influence the amount of radiation received by personnel considerably. Any solid material will absorb some nuclear radiation. Because of the very high penetrating power of neutrons and gamma rays, large amounts of material are required to provide significant protection. Dense materials such as lead, steel, concrete and earth offer the best protection against gamma rays. Materials such as water or concrete offer the best protection against neutrons. Earth is a fair neutron shield.

(3) A rough approximation of the percentage of the outside dose of initial gamma radiation and neutrons received by military personnel in various types of protection is shown in figure 11. Note that shielding against neutrons is more

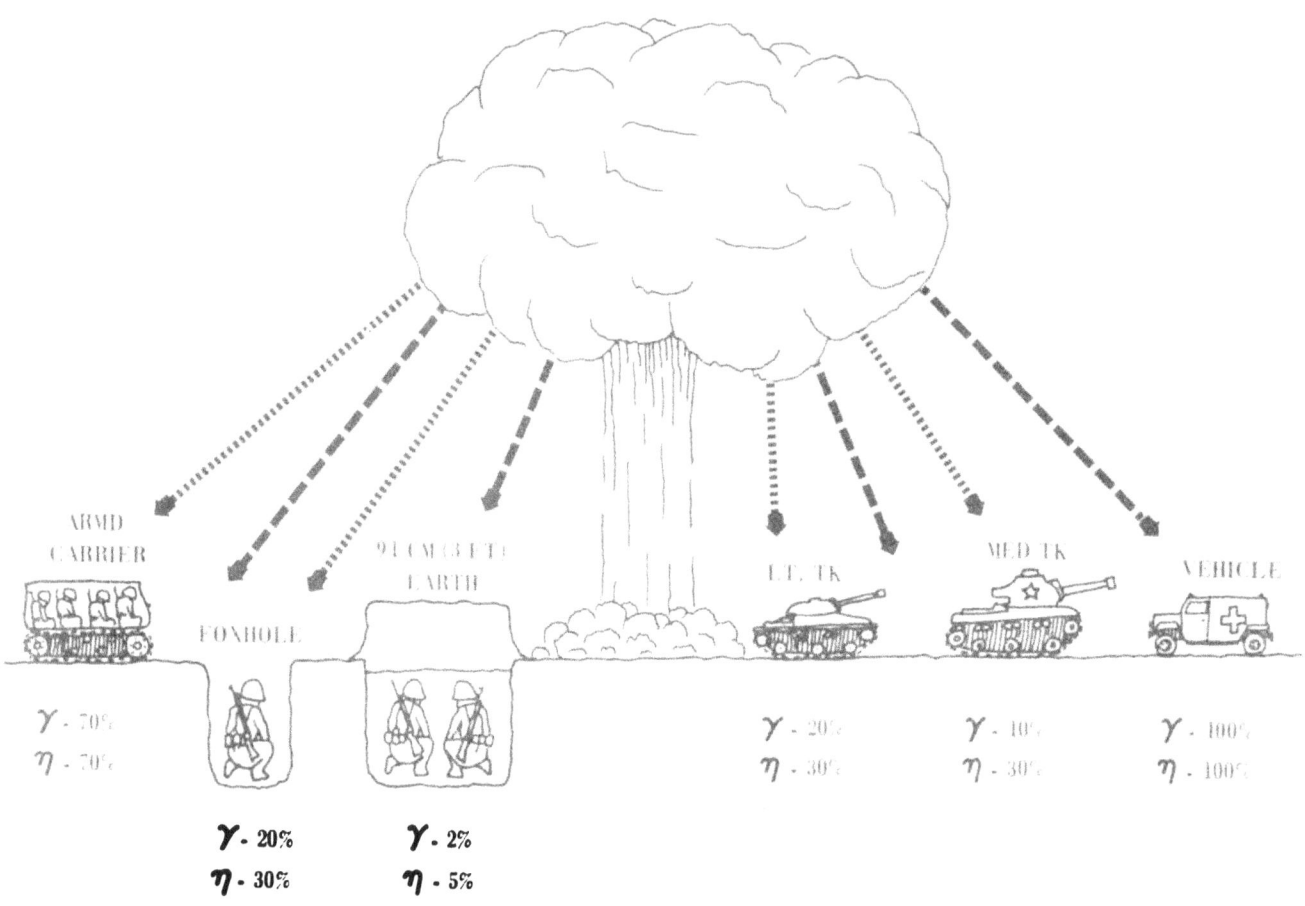

ARMD CARRIER

γ - 70%
η - 70%

FOXHOLE

γ - 20%
η - 30%

91 CM (3 FT) EARTH

γ - 2%
η - 5%

LT. TK

γ - 20%
η - 30%

MED TK

γ - 10%
η - 30%

VEHICLE

γ - 100%
η - 100%

Figure 11. Protection on battlefield against initial nuclear radiation.

difficult to achieve than is shielding against gamma rays.

b. *Residual Radiation.*

(1) *Protection against radiation.* Protection against residual nuclear radiation is a serious problem for the Medical Service for the following reasons:

(a) Early fallout may cover large areas of land with significantly high dose rates of gamma radiation. If there are large numbers of troops in these areas and if they are unprotected, the casualty production from the fallout may be far greater than that due to initial radiation, or to the thermal and blast effects.

(b) The fallout radiation hazard may persist for hours, days or even weeks after the detonation which produced it.

(c) Fallout will not only produce its own casualties but will also interfere with the treatment and evacuation of all other types of patients.

(2) *Types of radiation.* There are three kinds of radiation emitted from fallout—alpha and beta particles and gamma rays.

(a) The alpha hazard is of minor concern provided the radioactive fallout material is not deposited inside the body by ingestion or inhala-

tion. Even then, it is a hazard primarily in terms of years.

(b) The beta particles are of concern if the radioactive fallout material is deposited on the unprotected skin and remains for a prolonged period of time. The simple expedient of keeping one's clothing buttoned up and the early washing or wiping or brushing of oneself will do much to decrease the problem of beta burns.

(c) Because of its ability to penetrate tissue and cause serious radiation injury and travel great distances, it is the gamma radiation which forms the primary hazard in fallout.

(3) *Geometry of fallout radiation.* The whole-body gamma radiation hazard results from the total body exposure to radiation coming from some distance around an individual in a fallout area. As indicated in figure 12, essentially all of the dose to which the individual soldier may be exposed is a summation of gamma radiations from the contamination about him to a radius of approximately 100 meters (328 feet). Fifty percent of the dose comes from a circular area having a radius of approximately 10 meters (33 feet). He thus receives radiation from all directions, including from above. Gamma radiation is scattered in

50% OF DOSE FROM CIRCLE ABOUT 10 METERS IN RADIUS.

ESSENTIALLY ALL OF DOSE FROM CIRCLE ABOUT 100 METERS IN RADIUS.

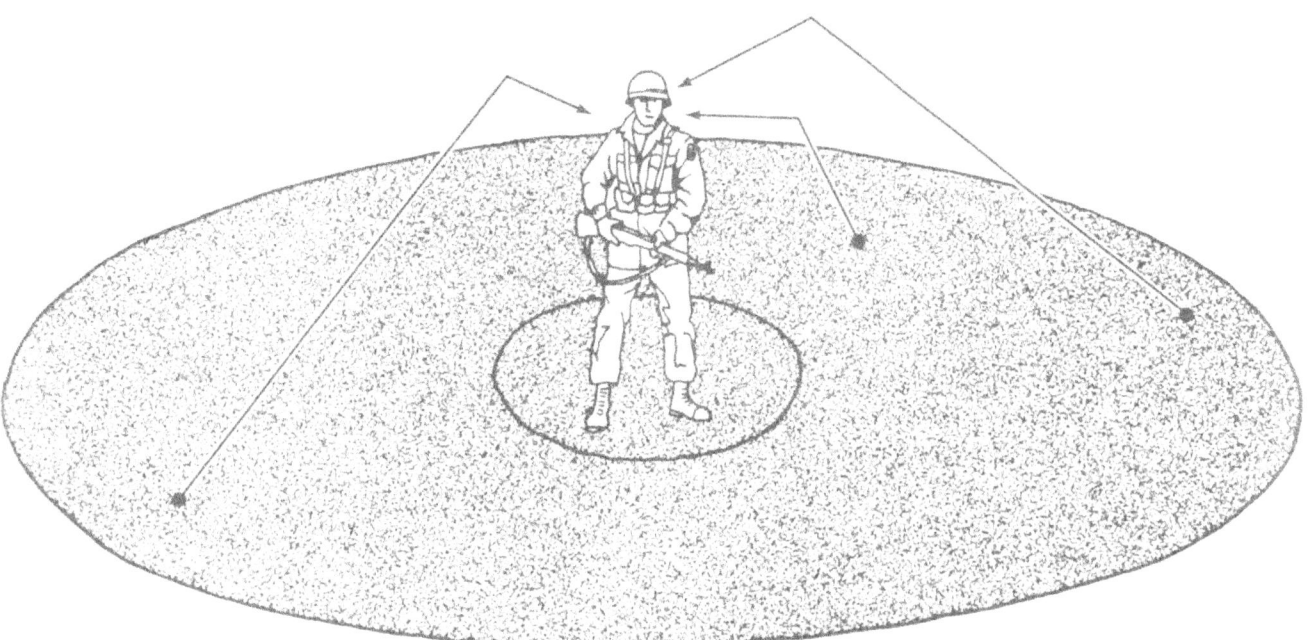

Figure 12. Geometry of fallout radiation.

the atmosphere just as other electromagnetic radiations, such as visible light. Therefore, a small but significant amount of gamma radiation can be received in the form of "Skyshine." If a soldier is in a foxhole, he will be shielded from most of the gamma radiation which comes from the surrounding ground. He will still receive the gamma from above unless he interposes some cover of earth (fig. 13). Extensive underground shelters will reduce the exposure to an absolute minimum.

(4) *Fallout decay curve.* Almost all fallout protective measures and operational decisions are ultimately based upon the concept of radioactive decay. All radioactive materials decay or lose radioactivity with the passage of time. Many of the fission products lose radioactivity very rapidly in the first few hours after a nuclear detonation. After a day or two, the rapidity of decay slows down considerably. This radioactive decay is illustrated in figure 14 (rate of decay is based on the standard decay constant 1.2). It can be seen that the early decay of the fission products is so rapid that at 7 hours after the detonation, any given quantity of fission product is emitting only 10 percent of the radiation emitted at 1 hour after the burst. This fact is sometimes expressed in a "rule of thumb" called the "Seven-ten" rule, which can be useful in estimating future dose rates in fallout areas. The "Seven-ten" rule simply states that for every sevenfold increase

in time, the dose rate decreases by a factor of 10^2. Time in this case is always expressed in hours after the burst, since it is the age of the fission products which determines the extent to which they have decayed radioactively.

c. *Fallout Shelter.* If a unit must remain in a fallout area, it can accomplish its mission and its personnel can survive only if adequate shelter is available. Fallout shelters provide protection against radiation through shielding. Many materials available on the battlefield offer substantial shielding against gamma radiation as shown in table 13. Generally, the denser or heavier the

Table 13. Shielding Potential of Common Materials

Material	Fallout gamma radiation
	½ Value layer thickness [3]
Steel	1.8 cm (.7″)
Concrete	5.6 cm (2.2″)
Earth	8.4 cm (3.3″)
Water	12.2 cm (4.8″)
Wood	22.4 cm (8.8″)

[3] If the radiation dose rate at 1 hr. after the explosion is taken as a reference point, than at 7 hrs. after the explosion the dose rate will have decreased to one-tenth; at 7 × 7 = 49 hours (or roughly 2 days) it will be one-hundredth; and at 7 × 7 × 7 = 348 hours (or roughly 2 weeks) the dose rate will be one-thousandth of that at 1 hr. after the burst.

[3] ½ Value Layer Thickness—Thickness of a given material which reduces the dose or dose rate to approximately one-half of that falling upon it.

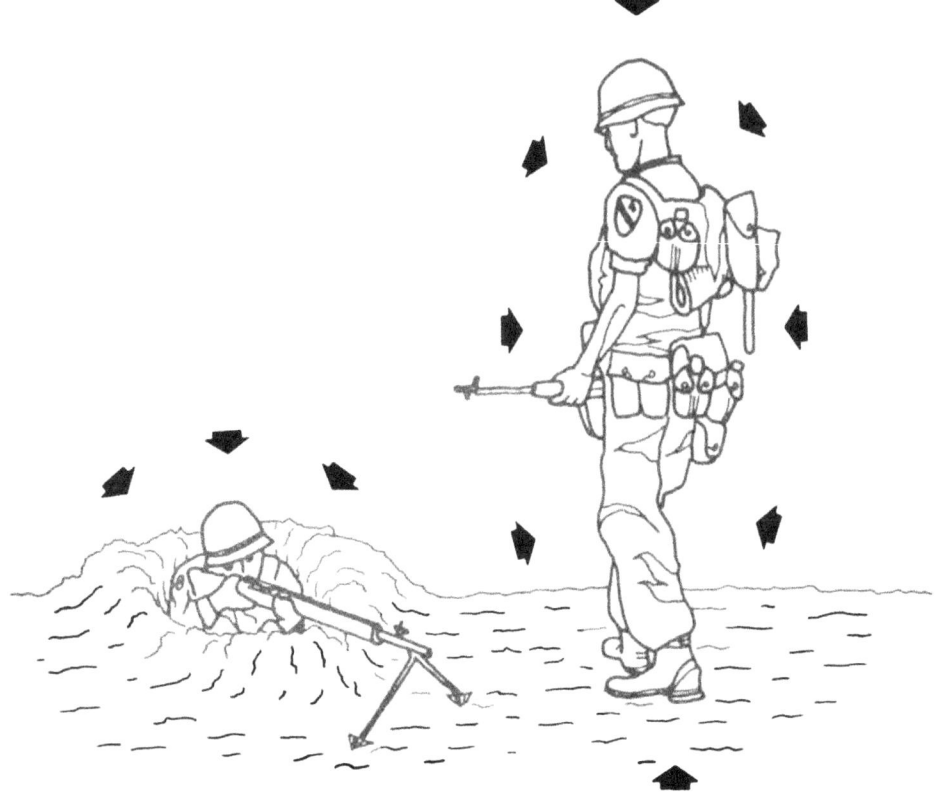

Figure 13. Geometry of fallout radiation—soldier in foxhole and in the open.

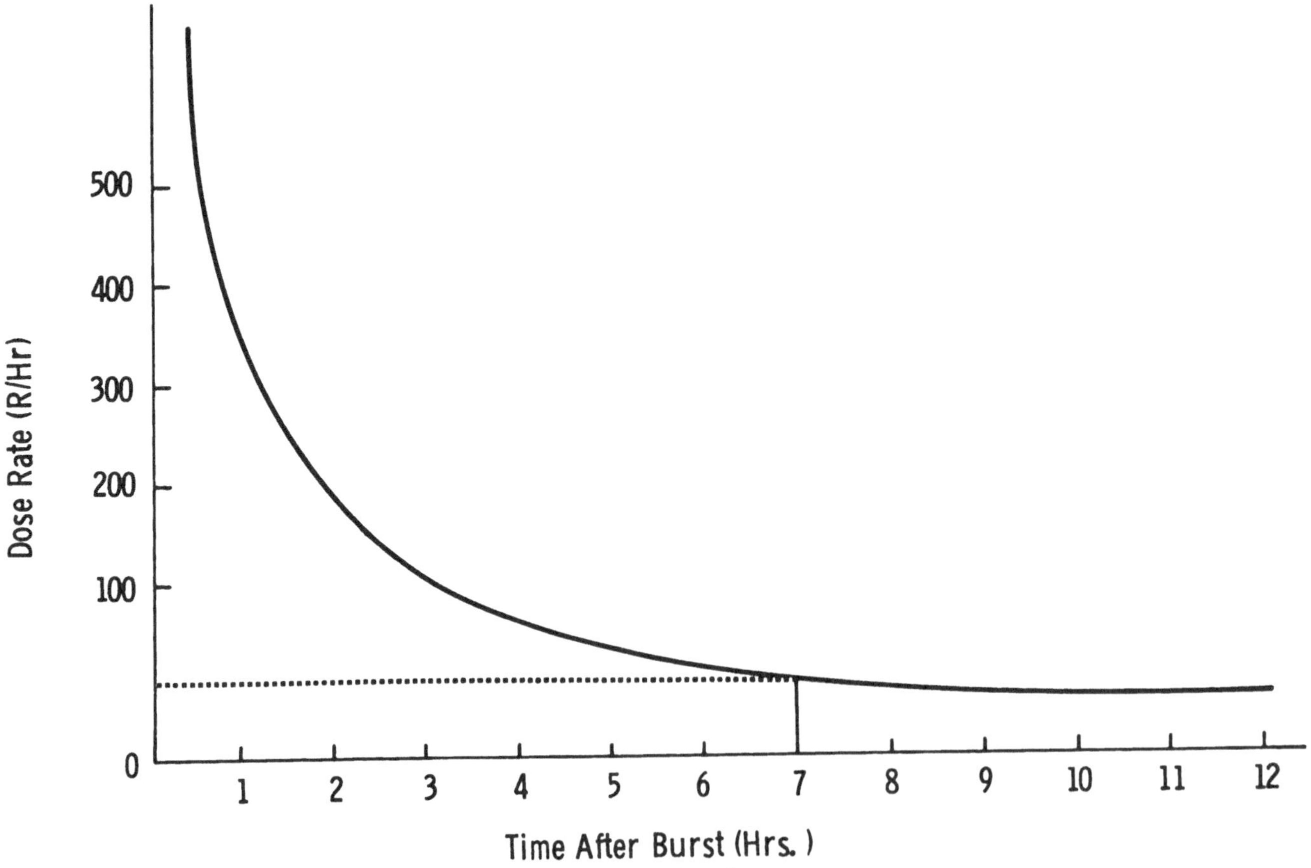

Figure 14. Radioactive decay.

material, the better shielding protection it offers against gamma radiation.

(1) The degree of protection afforded by a fallout shelter is usually expressed as a "protection factor," or a "transmission factor." The protection factor is simply the fraction of the available radiation dose which penetrates the shelter and reaches those inside compared to the radiation which would be received by an unprotected person. Thus a protection factor of 2 would indicate that an individual in the shelter would receive just half of the radiation dose he would receive if unprotected. A protection factor of 100 (associated with about six half-value thicknesses) indicates that only $\frac{1}{100}$ or 1 percent of the radiation dose reaches those inside. Transmission factors are expressed in percent or in decimals. Either refers to that fraction of the ambient unshielded dose which is received by personnel within the shelter. Fallout gamma transmission factors for some common shelter are shown in appendix D.

(2) In many cases it should be unnecessary to construct field expedient or any other type of fallout shelter since there are many such structures, and terrain features, available almost anywhere which may afford a degree of fallout protection. Tunnels, caves, culverts, overpasses, ditches, ravines and various manmade structures are examples of existing fallout shelter. The best possibility for existing shelter is basements. Figure 15 illustrates typical shelter protection provided by basements in different buildings. With little effort, windows can be sandbagged or covered with dirt from the outside to provide additional protection.

(3) It should become a matter of policy for mobile medical units to locate near existing shelter whenever possible. However, if a medical unit is already established, or must for some reason or another be established where no fallout shelter is available, then shelter must be constructed. Fortunately, elaborate shelters are not required, since they need be occupied continuously only for a day or two, with a maximum of about 3 days. There are a number of field expedients which will serve to save personnel and patients even though they may not be comfortable for those few days.

(4) The Dozer trench requires a minimum of engineer effort (fig. 16). A trench about 2.7 meters (9 feet) wide and 1.2 meter (4 feet) deep, as shown in figure 17, could be dug. About .6 meter (2 feet) length of trench for each person to be sheltered is required. Such trenches would probably reduce exposure of personnel lying on the floor to about 20–30 percent of what they would receive in the open. The engineers estimate that one dozer with its operator could cut 183 meters (600 feet) of such trench in 30 meter (100 foot) lengths in about 5 hours. Both protection and comfort can be improved from unit resources as time passes by digging the trench deeper, undercutting the walls, erecting tents over some portions of the trench, and providing flooring. In coordination with vigorous measures for individual and collective protection, dozer trenches should provide adequate fallout shelter for most fallout situations and provide it in a minimum of time and effort.

(5) The dug-in tents of a mobile hospital, as shown in figure 18, would provide more comfort and require less movement when fallout commenced than the dozer trench, however, it has two principal drawbacks. First, it offers far less radiation protection than the dozer trench and second, it requires considerably more in the way of engineer effort.

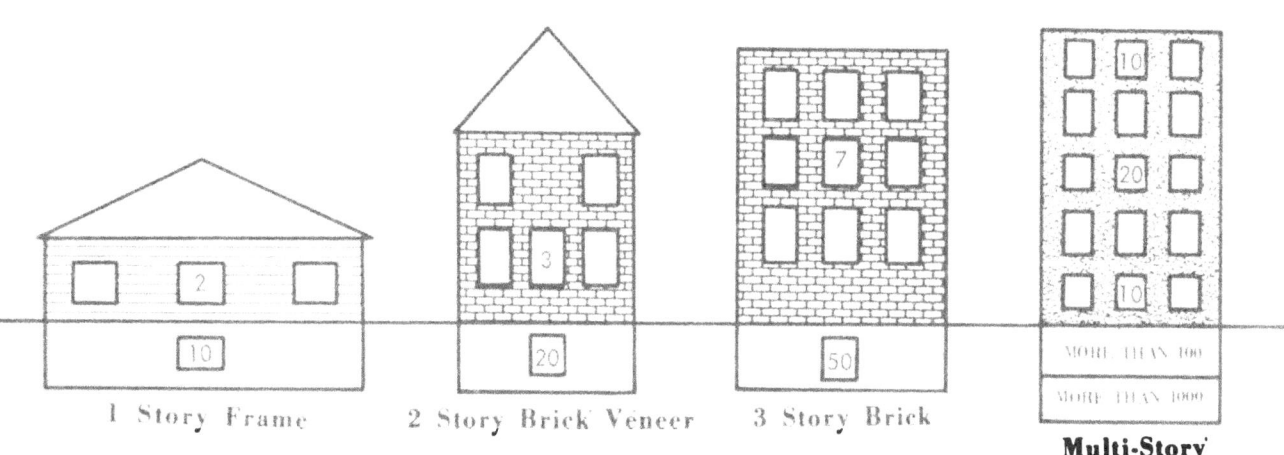

Figure 15. Approximate protection factor in buildings.

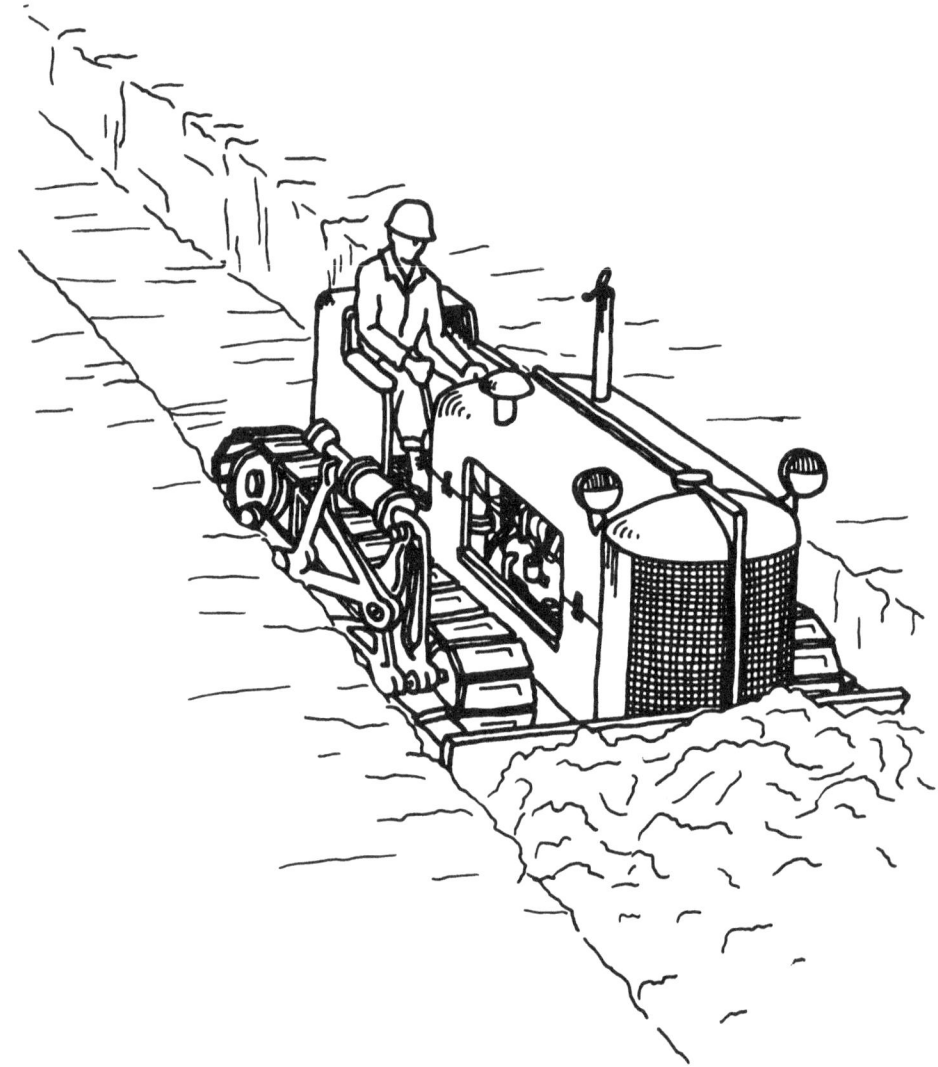

Figure 16. "Slot dozing" a trench.

(6) It is possible to build sandbag walls around the hospital tents as shown in figure 19 or lightly constructed buildings to provide fallout protection. Although sandbag walls to a height of 1.2 meter (4 feet) give significant protection (20–40 percent transmission factor) the effort required to achieved the protection is such that the measure is marginal in feasibility. Sandbagging is an effective means for supplementing other shelter by bolstering the shielding at weak spots, forming baffles, blocking open ends of trenches and covering windows and gaps.

(7) Another field expedient which is effective, combines the use of unit vehicles and dirt (fig. 20). *For example,* two general purpose large tents can be joined end-to-end and a shallow trench dug around them for the vehicles. The trench should be about 15 cm (6 inches) deep and the width of the vehicles. The dirt is piled carefully on the outside of the trench. An additional 15-cm (6

inch) trench is dug for the outer wheels of the vehicles. This combination of dirt and vehicles can give as much as 80 percent protection, if fallout contamination is collected and removed from inside the rectangle. Tent liners and ponchos can be used for this purpose. This expedient requires about 2 hours to build and can be occupied or evacuated in a matter of minutes. As with other expedient shelters, it should be constructed at the time the unit occupies the position.

(8) When no other shelter is available, medical units must prepare foxholes and slit trenches for patients and unit personnel. As time permits, these shelters must be improved by deepening, covering, undercutting, and sandbagging. Protection from nuclear radiation is required so that medical units can survive and function effectively. Suggested outline for fallout SOP for field medical units is shown in appendix C.

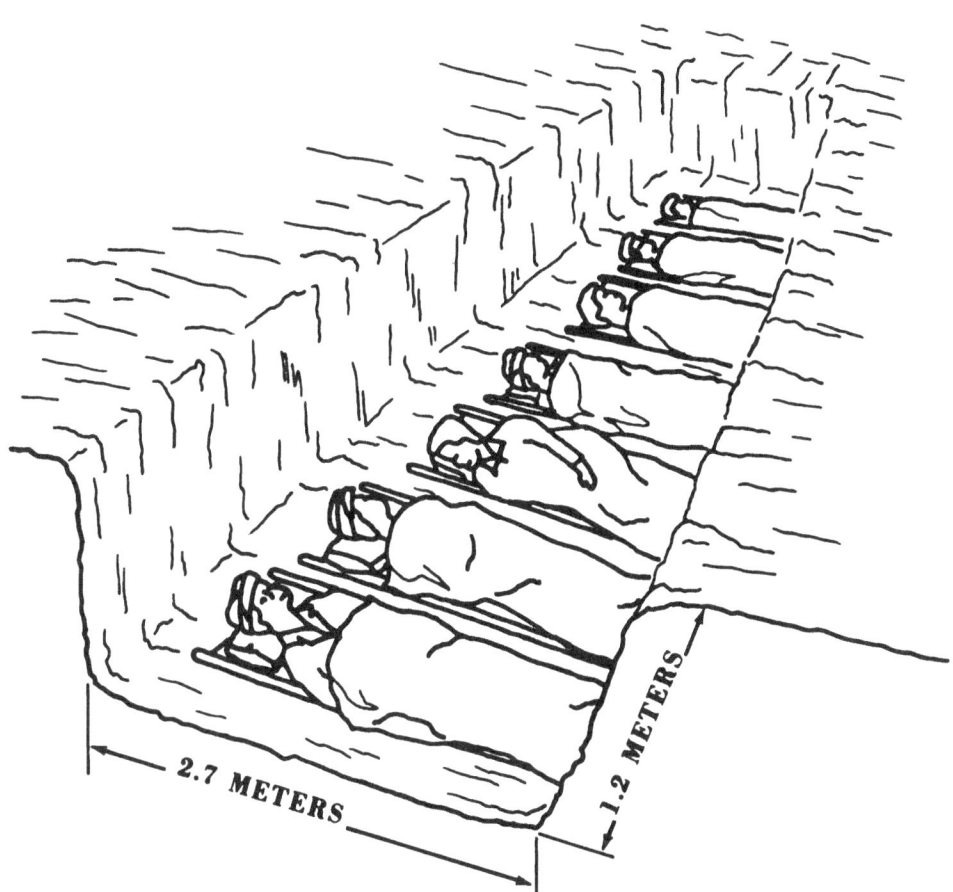

Figure 17. Dozer trench.

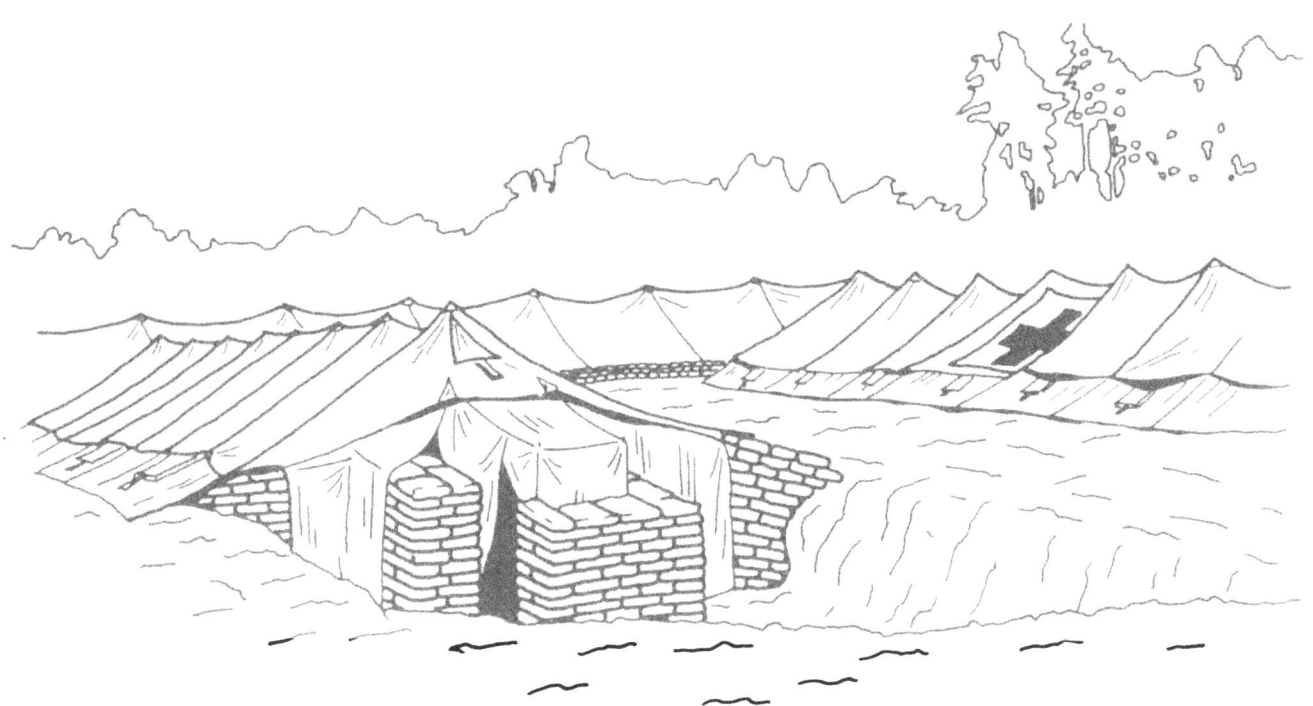

Figure 18. Dug-in tents.

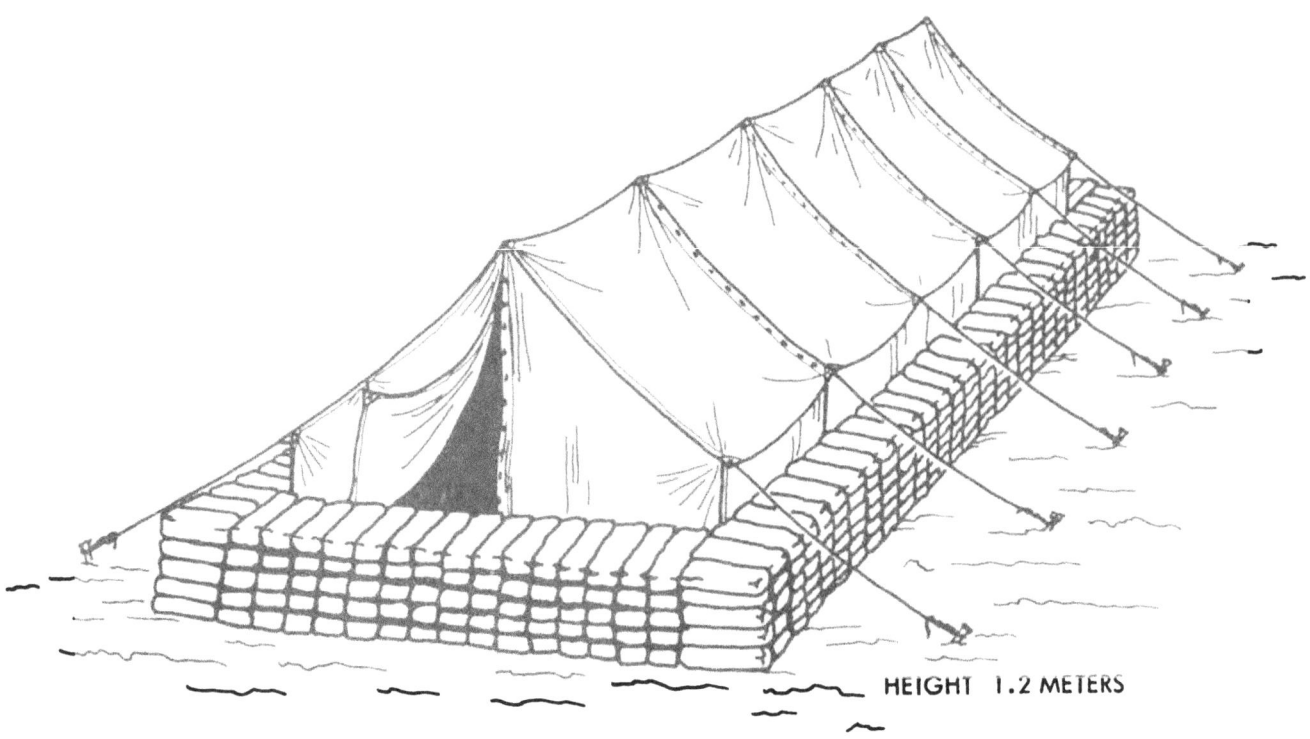

HEIGHT 1.2 METERS

Figure 19. Sandbag wall, bags placed crosswise.

25. Radioprotective Drugs

Several classes of chemical compounds have been shown to give varying degrees of protection against nuclear radiation injury in animals. The most effective compounds have been those containing sulfhydryl groups in their structure such as mercaptoethylamine (MEA) and 2-aminoethyl-isothiouronium (AET). If given a few minutes before radiation exposure, these substances may produce a protection factor of about 1.8 in experimental animals, i.e., the dose required to result in a specific mortality rate will be increased 1.8 times. However, the severe toxicity and short duration of action of drugs so far studied contra-indicate their use as radioprotective agents in humans.

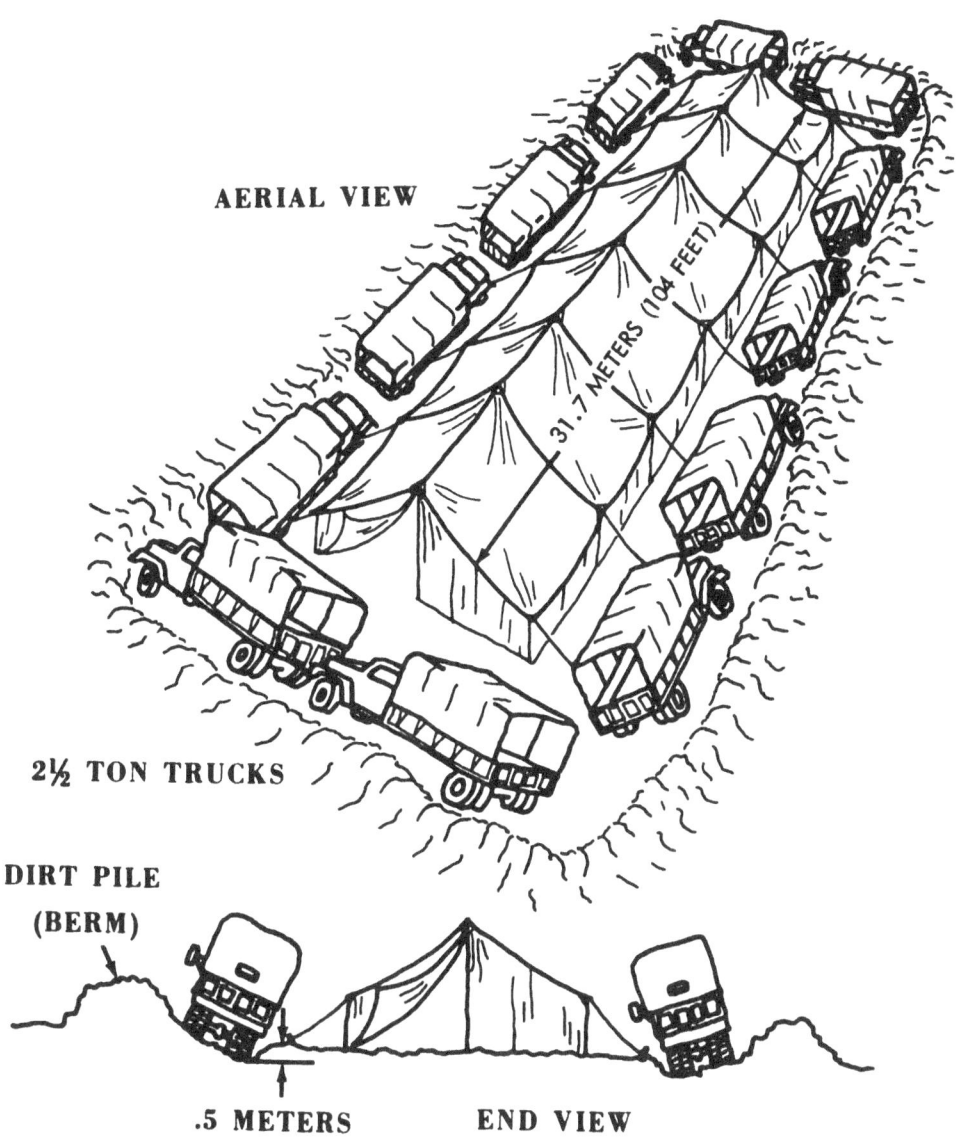

AERIAL VIEW

31.7 METERS (104 FEET)

2½ TON TRUCKS

DIRT PILE
(BERM)

.5 METERS   END VIEW

Figure 20. Fallout protection using vehicles and dirt.

CHAPTER 5

COMPARISON OF WEAPON EFFECTS

26. General

With the exception of residual radiation, the effects of a nuclear weapon occur simultaneously. It is, therefore, appropriate to discuss the integrated or combined effects of nuclear weapons. At any given location from ground zero, one can determine the effects which are acting simultaneously to produce casualties. In this chapter, the various weapon effects will be compared using the casualty criteria (table 14), as a basis. No attempt has been made to evaluate the synergistic effect of two or more casualty-producing mechanisms acting on a human target.

27. Governing Effect

a. Table 15 illustrates the relative importance of the three initial effects in the production of casualties as a function of range for various explosion yields. The areas included within the radii which represent the 4 hour (650 Rads) and 1 hour (3,000 Rads) sickness doses of ionizing radiation are relatively small and do not increase significantly as the weapon yield increases. Due to the manner in which ionizing radiation is degraded by distance, these radii of effects do not extend much beyond 2,500 meters (1.6 mile) even for a one megaton weapon. A thousand fold increase in yield extends the range only by a factor of 3. The radii for blast effects do show a proportionate increase with weapon yield. For serious missile injuries (50 percent probability) it can be seen that the range increases by a factor of 11 and for displacement injuries (50 percent probability of lethality) by a factor of 15. The thermal effects radii portray the distances within which second degree burns will occur on exposed skin and under the uniform. Table 14 demonstrates a dramatic increase in this range of 2° burns when the weapon yield is increased. For a 1 megaton weapon, 2° burns on exposed surfaces extends out to approximately 17,700 meters (11 miles) and includes an area of about 984 square kilometers (379 square miles). For 2° burns under the winter uniform (50 percent probability), the range is 8,370 meters (5.2 miles).

b. With the lower yield weapons, nuclear radiation injuries, compounded by mechanical injuries, will probably represent the predominant type of casualties. On the other hand, with the higher yield weapons, burns, wounds, and combinations thereof will represent the predominant types of injury from the initial effects. In a fallout area, nuclear radiation injuries will constitute the main medical problem.

Table 14. Casualty Criteria for Personnel Exposed to Prompt Effects

Effect	Criteria
Blast	3–5 psi—50% probability of serious wound from 10 gm. glass fragments in 3 meters of travel (Impact velocity 55 meters/sec).
	5–10 psi—50% probability of lethality from displacement in 3 meters of travel (impact velocity 8 meters/sec).
	22 psi— Foxhole collapse (>50% filling).
Thermal radiation	4–10 cal/cm²—2° burns on exposed surfaces.
	7.5–20 cal/cm²—50% probability of burns under summer uniform.
	10–26 cal/cm²—50% probability of burns under winter uniform.
Nuclear radiation	650 Rads—Nausea and vomiting within 4 hours.
	3000 Rads—Nausea and vomiting within 1 hour.

Table 15. Comparison of Weapon Effects (Airburst)

Casualty criteria	Yield			
	1 KT	10 KT	100 KT	1 MT
	(Distance in meters)			
50% probability of serious wounds (glass fragments).	740	1610	3860	8530
50% probability of lethality or displacement impact.	450	1130	2900	7080
Foxhole collapse (50% filling).	270	580	1260	2730
2° burns on exposed surfaces	805	2415	6440	17,700
2° burns—50% probability under summer uniform.	580	1480	3700	9330
2° burns—50% probability under winter uniform.	515	1200	3380	8370
650 Rads (Nausea and vomiting within 4 hours).	840	1290	1770	2570
3000 Rads (Nausea and vomiting within 1 hour).	580	970	1530	2090

CHAPTER 6

PSYCHOLOGICAL EFFECTS

28. General

Although it is possible to estimate roughly the number of injured and dead which would result from the thermal, blast, and radiation effects of a nuclear weapon used in combat, it is much more difficult to predict the numbers and types of psychiatric patients. It is generally felt that the acute psychological problems which would occur in such circumstances would be essentially the same as those seen in other combat situations, and that the treatment methods which have been developed as a result of experience in past wars would be appropriate.

29. Clinical Signs and Symptoms

a. The primary psychological abnormality which develops in severe stress or disaster situations is a transient, fluid state of emotional disruption. This occurs when an individual cannot cope with the danger presented to him by his environment. Its major features are fear and the results therefrom. The fear develops largely from the individual's inability to make meaningful decisions or initiate purposeful actions; and as a result, even minor decisions become difficult to make. A vicious circle of Fear-Inaction-Fear may ensue, and the individual involved may become ineffective. This may vary in degree all the way from very mild to complete helplessness.

b. Panic, defined as frantic, irrational behavior associated with real or supposed trapping, probably would be rare, since it has been found to be rare in other disaster situations.

c. Chronic mental disease, either psychotic or neurotic, also would probably be rare. This again reflects the finding that these reactions are not commonly seen in disaster situations.

d. Precipitous flight with direction and purpose is not panic and should be considered a useful and practical response to the situation.

e. Characteristic disturbances which would include: stunned mute behavior, uncontrolled flight, tearful helplessness, apathetic depressed states, inappropriate activity, increased tension, or preoccupation with somatic representations. These

disturbances can last for minutes, hours, days, or sometimes weeks. Fortunately, people with the milder and shorter reactions are in the majority.

f. A major characteristic of these patients is their suggestibility, and it is this which forms the basis for the treatment methods described in paragraph 30.

g. The frequency and severity of the psychological disturbances vary with several factors—

(1) *Intensity and severity of stress.* Stressful situations of brief duration are rather easily tolerated, and recovery of individuals with mild degrees of mental disruption under these circumstances is rapid. If stressful situations follow one another rapidly, or if any one of them is of long duration, then the probability of the occurrence of more severe psychological reactions of longer duration increases.

(2) *Degree of personal involvement.* If an individual has a "close call" or if he sees close friends or relatives severely injured, his reaction will be more severe than if he remains "relatively" remote from danger.

(3) *Degree of training.* This is the most important factor in that it is the one which is most easy to modify. A well-trained individual, who can react instinctively to dangerous situations and initiate appropriate actions, will develop a minimum of incapacitating fear. The fear he does develop will, if anything, help him, since it will be an integral part of a reaction of increased awareness or alertness allowing more efficient fight or flight.

(4) *Degree of warning.* This is closely related to (3) above. Warning helps a trained person to prepare. He can initiate proper actions early. For an untrained person, the effect will be variable. If fear of incapacitating degree occurs, then the warning may well result in more harm or danger. If the fear is not incapacitating, then the untrained person who cannot react automatically to initiate proper actions may be able to utilize the time to improvise appropriate action. Whatever time he has to do this will help.

(5) *Presence or absence of leadership.* In a group in a disaster situation, a few individuals will emerge as leaders. These may not be the appointed leaders, although in a military unit this is usually not the case unless the appointed or regular leaders become ineffective or are lost. When effective leadership is available, the group will fare much better than when there is none.

(6) *Group identification.* This is a particularly important factor for the military. If group or unit integrity is preserved, the individuals in the unit will do much better. Also, those individuals with mild psychological disruptions will recover faster if they can remain with or close to their unit, thus retaining their personal relationship as a member of the unit.

30. Treatment

a. The psychological disorders described above do not require elaborate treatment. The best treatment is that which is simple, direct, and immediate. It should be done as far forward as possible, preferably within the unit to which the individual belongs. If this is not possible, then it should be started as soon as possible and in a medical facility close to the individual's unit. Evacuation to distant medical facilities is contraindicated, as this tends to make the psychological problems worse by severing the patient's relationship to his group or unit and by introducing the element of "secondary gain" with the removal of the patient from danger.

b. The treatment consists of—

(1) *Reassurance and suggestion that the situation will improve.* These people are suggestible early in their disruptive phase and simple reassurance using a positive, direct approach is usually successful. The patient should be made to feel that he has an excellent chance for recovery, which, in general, is true.

(2) *Rest with removal from immediate danger.* A short period of rest in a safe area is of great benefit.

(3) *Ventilation.* Retention of fear and anxiety by the more severely incapacitated frequently blocks effective communication. When the patient expresses his feelings, this tends to remove this block. This communication is essential before the individual can recover enough to rejoin the activities of his "group" or unit.

c. Psychiatrists are not always available to participate in the overall treatment of such patients. Therefore, all medical officers and their staff should be familiar with these principles for managing the psychological problems arising from such disasters. The success of their action will depend largely on how well the line commanders understand the program of managing this problem, since in a great degree the practical therapy of the mildly affected will be, in fact, the positive leadership actions taken by commanders.

31. Prevention

The most important preventive factor is intensive training. The end result of proper training is less fear and more prompt effective action. Action relieves tension, so that the fear response is less likely to become severe or incapacitating. Fear may not even develop to the point where the individual is aware of it. Various other factors which contribute to prevention include discipline, morale, good leadership, and promotion of group identification. The beneficial results of effective command cannot be overemphasized.

CHAPTER 7

MEDICAL MANAGEMENT OF PATIENTS IN NUCLEAR WARFARE

32. General

The successful early management of patients depends upon the exercise of sound judgment in the following basic areas:

a. Medical sorting of patients (Triage).

b. Treatment. This should be directed toward providing maximum benefit to the greatest number under the circumstances while avoiding any procedure which would unwarrantably reduce the patient's ability to care for himself.

c. Utilization of medical service personnel. Medically trained individuals must be used efficiently and should not be diverted to first aid, rescue, transportation, or nonmedical labor functions.

d. Flexibility of the supporting medical facility to respond and adapt to rapidly changing circumstances.

e. Rigorous supply conservation.

f. Evacuation of casualties.

g. Planning and training. Preparation for the management of patients in nuclear warfare must be based on a knowledge of nuclear weapons effects and sound medical practices. Training must be practical rather than theoretical.

33. Medical Sorting

a. Medical sorting or triage is the key to the effective management of large numbers of sick and wounded. It includes the immediate classification of patients according to type and seriousness of injury and likelihood of survival, and the establishment of priorities for treatment and evacuation to assure medical care of the greatest benefit to the largest number. Sorting permits the orderly, timely, and efficient utilization of available medical means. It is a continuous process, carried out at each echelon of medical care as patients are evacuated rearward. The critical importance of sorting demands that medical officers assigned this responsibility be selected on the basis of mature professional judgment.

b. Criteria for the classification of patients will vary with the military situation, the patient load, and the capability of the medical unit involved.

The following is a classification of patients according to their need for medical care and chance for survival:

(1) *Patients requiring* **Minimal** *treatment:* Those who may be returned to duty include those who have: 1) small lacerations or contusions, 2) simple fractures of small bones, 3) second-degree burns of less than 10 percent extent but not involving face or hands, or who have received, 4) short term body ionizing radiation doses of 100 to 150 rads. The second group includes noneffective persons who need minimal nursing care for: 1) disabling minor fractures; 2) burns of the face or hands which interfere with the person's ability to care for himself; 3) moderate neuropsychiatric disorders, or, 4) early symptoms of nausea and vomiting due to short term wholebody ionizing radiation doses of 150 rads or less. These patients truly have no priority for treatment but in practice would receive some treatment when first seen. Ordinarily, their wounds and diseases would be such that the treatment they receive while being sorted is all the treatment they would require, and they could then be returned to duty or sent to a facility for minimal nursing care. This group could constitute up to 40 percent of the total injured.

(2) *Patients requiring* **Immediate Care**. Included as patients requiring immediate care are those with: 1) hemorrhage from an easily accessible site, 2) rapidly correctible mechanical respiratory defects, 3) severe crushing wounds of the extremities, 4) incomplete amputations, 5) severe lacerations with open fractures of major bones, and 6) severe burns of the face and upper respiratory tract necessitating tracheotomy. The patients in group 2 will be given the highest priority for surgical treatment because a relatively short procedure could save life or limb. More definitive surgery would be delayed to a later date. An increased rate of complications and permanent disability would have to be accepted. This group is expected to comprise about 20 percent of the total injured.

(3) *Patients whose surgical treatment may*

be Delayed. Persons whose surgical treatment can be delayed without immediate jeopardy to life include those with: 1) simple closed fractures of major bones, 2) moderate lacerations without extensive bleeding, 3) second-degree burns of 10 percent to 25 percent and third-degree burns of 10 percent to 15 percent of the body surface (after body fluid levels have been stabilized), and 4) noncritical central-nervous-system injuries. This group is composed of patients for whom a delay in treatment might lead to complications but whose lives would not be unduly jeopardized by delay. The amount of delay between wounding and surgery for this group depends on the total number of patients with higher priorities who need treatment and the medical facilities available. This group may comprise about 20 percent of all injured.

(4) *Patients whose treatment would be on an extended delayed basis (Expectant).* These patients include those with: 1) critical injuries of the central nervous system or respiratory system, 2) penetrating abdominal wounds, 3) multiple severe injuries, 4) severe burns of large areas (30 percent or above), or 5) known lethal or supralethal doses of total body radiation. The treatment for group 4 patients would consist of that resuscitation and emergency medical treatment which the available facilities, total supplies, and number of professional personnel permit. They would have the lowest priority for surgery because the operative procedures required would be time consuming and technically complicated, so that an operation on one of these patients would theoretically jeopardize the lives of several in other higher priority groups. The more rapidly patients in other treatment categories are treated and moved, the sooner more definitive treatment could be started on the injured in category 4. It is anticipated that this group will comprise about 20 percent of all injured.

c. The percentages noted above for each classification may vary considerably in a specific instance during nuclear warfare, depending on a multitude of factors including the physical environment, orientation of the personnel, weapon employment, time of day, presence or absence of fallout, and many other variables.

34. Handling the Radioactively Contaminated Patient

a. Patients who have been in fallout areas may have varying amounts of radioactive contamination on their skin and clothing. The contamination will be in the form of fission products which have become absorbed on the surfaces of dirt or dust particles of varying sizes. The patient himself will not be radioactive, but he will suffer radiation injury (beta burns) from the contamination unless it is removed early. In addition, as the patient is handled, much of the contamination will be scattered about, contaminating other people and the surroundings. The objective of proper decontamination is to control the removal of this hazardous material from patients, restricting it to defined areas. This will allow proper handling of contaminated equipment and clothing and will reduce the hazard to other personnel.

b. It is important to bear in mind the distinction between contaminated patients and radiation injured patients. Patients who have received substantial doses of radiation and who subsequently exhibit clinical manifestations of the acute radiation syndrome are not necessarily contaminated. Likewise, patients who are contaminated have not necessarily received substantial doses of radiation. Mere exposure to radiation does not result in a contaminated casualty. Only when substances emitting radiation are deposited upon, or become attached to, the patient or his clothing is the patient radiologically contaminated.

c. The presence of fallout contamination upon a patient represents by far a greater hazard to the patient himself than it does to the personnel caring for him. The duration of the exposure, the quantity of contact contamination, the distance between the source and those exposed, and the geometry of the radiation exposure all combine to maximize the danger to the patient while minimizing that to those around. Further, if the medical facility which receives the contaminated patients is itself in a fallout area, the high gamma environment and its threat to all patients and medical personnel would far outweigh any hazards from handling contaminated patients.

d. Fear that the gathering of large numbers of heavily contaminated patients in or around a medical facility is hazardous is unfounded. The only hazard from radioactive contamination which can cause injury at any distance in air is gamma radiation. It would be very difficult to get enough patients crowded together to constitute a significant gamma hazard. If all the radioactive contamination from many heavily contaminated patients was collected in one small area of a few square meters, a minor hazard could result, but the patients themselves will not present a gamma hazard.

e. The major hazard associated with handling contaminated patients is the possibility of beta burns caused by transfer of the radioactive material from the patients to the unprotected skin surfaces of other personnel. Though this hazard is not a lethal one, it could result in the incapacitation of medical personnel from the burns if the material is not removed from their skin.

f. In order to handle the radiologically contaminated patients properly, it is first necessary to detect contaminated patients. The only way to detect radioactive contamination is by proper monitoring with radiac instruments. Since the levels of radiation to be dealt with are rather low and the governing hazard is beta radiation, a Geiger-Mueller counter such as the AN/PDR–27 should be used to monitor incoming patients for contamination. As a general rule, if the reading is twice current background radiation or higher, the patient should be considered contaminated.

g. Incoming patients should be monitored at any time there is any reason to believe that contaminated patients are arriving at the medical facility. (Possible indications: reports from ambulance drivers, messages from another hospital or a headquarters, sighting of a nuclear burst or cloud.) Otherwise, patients may be "spot checked" every 15 minutes or every five or six patients. This monitoring need not be carried out at a great distance from the medical facility. It can be accomplished within or just outside the admission area. The only requirement is that it be done if at all possible prior to admission of the patient to the facility. Once it has been confirmed that the patient is contaminated, decontamination is easily accomplished. The simple removal of all outer clothing and a brief washing or brushing of the exposed skin surfaces will achieve a high degree of decontamination without subjecting the patient to the trauma of vigorous bathing and showering. These simple tasks can be accomplished prior to admission or later on the ward or elsewhere in the medical facility depending upon the condition of the patient. *The radiological contamination of the patient should not be allowed to interfere with immediate life saving treatment or the best possible medical care.* However, whenever decontamination of a patient is done, the material removed results in contamination of another area. If a patient is brushed or washed off, all the material removed must be collected and removed from the medical facility. Even though the quantities of radioactive material on one patient may be small, the uncontrolled removal of contamination from large numbers of patients could result in hazardous accumulations of materials in hospital facilities. Problems can arise as a result of trying to decontaminate seriously injured patients who require extensive resuscitative and surgical treatment without delay. It may be necessary to accept a certain amount of contamination in the treatment facilities, during the care of such patients. At intervals when possible, thorough cleaning of the areas will have to be done.

h. It is desirable for those handling patients before or during their decontamination to wear gloves. Any gloves will help, but rubber gloves are preferable. Monitors should supervise disposition of contaminated clothing and equipment, and all staff personnel must emphasize normal hygiene, such as washing hands and face.

i. Whenever a contaminated patient is admitted to the facility prior to complete decontamination, his records should be clearly marked to indicate that he is contaminated. Any suitable code word may be used, such as "RADCON," so long as personnel who come in contact with the patient understand its meaning. After incompletely decontaminated patients have been admitted, monitors should make followup rounds of clinics and wards. When the decontamination of the patient has been completed within the facility, and the monitor verifies this, the monitor should line out the code word and enter the word "clear" along with the date and his initials on the medical record. The patient need receive no special treatment or handling thereafter for reasons of radiological contamination.

j. The receipt of contaminated patients by a medical facility need not require the declaration of any alert or special "condition" throughout the facility. Only the few people who come in direct contact with the patient prior to decontamination need be concerned. Monitors who detect the contamination should notify those in the admission area and those in the supply section who may handle contaminated clothing and equipment. Others in the facility who come in contact with the patient prior to completion of decontamination will be alerted to the extent necessary by the coded entry on the patient's attached record. These are the only members of the staff who need be concerned about the situation (app B).

CHAPTER 8

PUBLIC HEALTH AND PREVENTIVE MEDICINE

35. General

In this chapter problems in the field of public health and preventive medicine following the use of nuclear weapons will be considered. Combat is rarely in uninhabited areas, and the disruptive effects of combat operations on civilian populations and facilities can be very severe. These can in turn markedly affect military operations in an area.

36. Determining Factors

a. Certain factors are of prime importance in determining the nature and severity of the effects.

    (1) Population density.

    (2) Degree of urbanization.

    (3) Degree of industrialization.

    (4) Availability of food supplies.

    (5) Availability of water.

    (6) Climate.

b. Other considerations such as the moral and legal requirements to defend and assist allies, including civilians, will also affect military medical planning and operations.

c. Finally, the manner and situation in which nuclear weapons are used are of importance. If a single weapon is detonated in an area which has otherwise been spared devastation and in which there is social stability, the results will be far less serious than if one or more weapons are used in areas where prolonged or severe combat has already disrupted the various elements which make up a stable society. At Hiroshima and Nagasaki, which are excellent samples of the first type of situation, the survivors who could get away were able to obtain food, shelter, and care from surrounding intact areas. With prolonged combat, such intact areas probably would not be available, and the result would be no food, shelter, or care for any survivors. Such a picture is a more realistic prediction of the status of civilian populations in a theater in which prolonged combat with nuclear weapons was occurring. There would be nearly complete breakdown of social order and a complete lack of effective medical care. This would include preventive medicine and public health functions and facilities.

37. Disease Incidence

a. Without preventive medicine and public health capabilities, considerably increased incidence and morbidity from diseases of all types would follow. Certain diseases would predominate in incidence, depending upon the geographical areas involved and the endemic diseases present.

b. In urban areas in temperature climates such as North America and Europe several diseases are epidemic threats.

    (1) Dysenteries due to a variety of pathogens.

    (2) Rickettsial diseases, particularly typhus and scrub typhus.

    (3) Hepatitis.

    (4) Plague.

    (5) Tuberculosis.

    (6) Venereal diseases of all types.

c. In many parts of the world, in addition to the diseases listed above, malaria and cholera are threats.

d. There are several reasons for the increased risk of disease.

    (1) Crowding of surviving populations with limited sanitary facilities such as was seen in Europe at the end of World War II.

    (2) Lack of immunization facilities with resultant increases in the susceptible fraction of a given population.

    (3) Lack of vector and pest control.

    (4) Effect of irradiation on susceptibility to infection: With high levels of fallout covering wide areas, a large number of people would sustain sublethal whole-body doses of irradiation. The interaction of such types of irradiation with infectious states is not clear, but it is quite possible that the result would be uncovering of latent infection and decreased resistance to infection. This would result in an increased incidence of disease.

    (5) Upsets in ecological balance and host-

parasite relationship following the use of nuclear weapons: Different classes and orders of animals have marked differences in sensitivity to irradiation. Insects, for example, are much more resistant than are vertebrates. It is conceivable that the normal balance between insects and birds which prey upon them in a given area would be severely upset resulting in a marked overgrowth of the insects. If these included vectors of disease or insects which could destroy vegetation, there would be serious increases in disease hazards or serious destruction of food crops.

CHAPTER 9

OPERATIONAL PROBLEMS FOR MEDICAL PERSONNEL

38. General

a. Successful medical operations on the nuclear battlefield require timely and knowledgeable decisions. Surgeons, unit commanders, and staff officers must understand the problems imposed by nuclear environment. Decisions concerning how to minimize the effect of blast, thermal radiation, and initial nuclear radiation must be made in advance of the event. Those things which must be accomplished to minimize the prompt effects are simple and straightforward—

(1) Dispersion.

(2) Shelter.

(3) Avoidance of likely nuclear targets.

Once the bomb has exploded, there is little one can do to alter the number of casualties which may be produced.

b. In the case of fallout, things are quite different. The fallout radiation hazard may cover thousands of square kilometers and persist for many hours or even days. There is not only time to make decisions, but a vital necessity that they be made. These decisions will not merely affect the outcome, they will determine it.

39. Unit Survival and Performance of Mission in Fallout

Medical personnel and medical units generally will be faced with two primary problems when operating in a significant local fallout situation. The first of these is unit survival and the second is the performance of the mission.

a. Unit Survival. To survive in a fallout situation the existence of the hazard must first be recognized. Information pertaining to the location and intensity of radiologically contaminated areas may be provided the medical units by higher headquarters. In all probability, however, medical units will receive little warning of impending fallout. Even if this information were available in sufficient time to the medical unit, it would not necessarily represent the key to action. It will be the unit CBR team which will determine the absence or presence of fallout, collect and analyze the radiac data, and assist the medical commander

in formulating decisions as to actions necessary for unit survival.

b. Radiac Instruments. Radiac instruments are a basic requirement for dealing with the fallout radiation hazard. Without them there is no means to evaluate the hazard or know that one exists. Some types of radiac instruments currently provided Army units are shown in table 16.

c. Defensive Action Procedures. Once the hazard is recognized, the medical unit must then be prepared to take defensive action by moving, if at all possible, to prepared shelter areas. Where the medical unit does not occupy buildings with basements, caves or other underground structures and finds itself under tentage, the field expedients as described in paragraph 24 must be used. The construction of these field expedients must have been done in advance rather than after the occurrence of fallout. A medical unit commander should notify higher headquarters of the onset of fallout in his area by the most expeditious means, and if possible, patients should be diverted from treatment units operating in the contaminated areas. Normal evacuation should be resumed as soon as the radiological situation permits.

d. Performance of Mission—Shelter Operations.

(1) *Patients.* Should evacuation of patients to a shelter area become necessary, professional care may have to revert to simple supportive measures and surgical procedures limited to those urgently required to save life and possibly limb.

(2) *Control.* Personnel should remain in shelter during fallout unless specifically authorized to leave shelter sooner to perform a specific task. Prior to authorized departure from shelter during fallout, the departing individual should be briefed by monitoring personnel on precautions to be observed, and have an IM–93 dosimeter attached to his clothing. When the individual returns, he must brush himself off, and the monitor should read the IM–93 and record his exposure on the unit *Radiation Dose Status Chart.* Rotation of personnel who leave shelter should be practiced.

(3) *Communications.* Telephonic or radio communication between unit headquarters and

Table 16. Radiac Instruments

Instrument	Range	Function	Detection capability	Miscellaneous information
Radiac Set AN/PDR–27.	0–500 mrad/hr	Monitoring (Personnel, food, water, and equipment).	Gamma Beta (detection only).	GM type dose rate instrument; Battery operated; Weight 8 lbs; Accuracy ±20%; 11 per Med Bn Inf and Armored Div; 2 per Med Co Airborne Div; 2 per hosp with less than 400 beds; 3 per hosp with 400–750 beds; 1 per medical section in any unit.
Radiacmeter IM–174A/PD.	0–500 rad/hr	Survey Monitoring (Areas only; not suitable for personnel food, water, and equipment).	Gamma _____	Ion-chamber type dose rate instrument; Battery operated; Weight 3¾ lb; Accuracy ±20%; 2 per hosp; 1 per platoon.
Radiacmeter IM–93/UD.	0–600 rad	Dosimeter _____	Gamma X-ray.	Total dose instrument; self-reading; Weight 2 oz; Requires electrostatic charger (PP–1578A/PD); Calibration accuracy ±5%; 2 per platoon.
Radiacmeter AN/PDR–60.	0–2,000,000 CPM/59 cm² 0–2 rad/hr	Survey Monitoring.	Alpha Gamma.	Scintillation and GM type dose rate instrument. Battery operated. Weight 6 lb. Basis of issue: As required by Nuclear Emergency Teams.

principal shelter areas, including patient shelter areas, must be maintained. Noise should be kept to a minimum throughout the unit area to facilitate voice communication. A public address system would be a valuable asset for this purpose. Runners should be employed for communication only when the urgency of the message is commensurate with the exposure to be suffered by the individual.

(4) *Advance planning.* Problems of human waste disposal and disposal of bodies will probably require a local decision which will vary with the circumstances faced at the time. However, prior thought in planning for these events by varying type of units may make the decision more easily attainable at the time of the event. The placement of varying categories of patients should evacuation to a shelter area become necessary may relieve the need for the mass movement of the critically injured (lowest priority) patient into the area of maximum shelter.

(5) *Dosimetry.* Unit CBR personnel should make radiation background readings in the open. At least two IM–93 tactical dosimeters should be located outside the unit headquarters in an unsheltered location approximately 91 centimeters (3 feet) above the ground. Readings from these instruments should be taken at least twice daily. Dosimeters must be recharged at least weekly and should be protected from direct contamination. Following the passage of the fallout peak, a survey of the unit area should be made and findings reported to higher headquarters. "Hot spots" should be properly marked on the ground, and avoided. The radiological situation inside the shelter should be determined early. While appendix D gives transmission factors of typical shelters, the actual protection should be determined with the tactical dose rate meters. The unit CBR personnel may be able to obtain outside readings remotely by using field glasses or pulleys.

(6) *Food and water.* Rations of the C-type or other packaged types for all anticipated shelter occupants should be distributed to the shelter areas.

Water trailers or vehicles and fuel sources should be placed where they are accessible with a minimum of radiation exposure to occupants of shelters. Filled 5-gallon cans of water should be used in areas remote to the above water sources. Individual canteens should be refilled as soon as used.

(7) *Film protection.* Unexposed X-ray film should be placed in a hole in the shelter floor.

The hole should be at least 91 centimeters (3 feet) deep and covered with two layers of sandbags or the equivalent in loose earth. A niche in the wall of a below-ground shelter would provide similar protection.

40. Contamination and Decontamination of Food, Water, Personnel, and Material

a. Food and Water. After a nuclear attack, in addition to protection from external radiation exposure, it is important that personnel in the fallout area be protected from internal radiation exposure due to the ingestion of radioactively contaminated food and water. Although the ingestion of contaminated food and water is not an immediate threat to survival, there is the possibility of late somatic and genetic effects. It is essential, therefore, that every effort be made to remove the radioactive material from food and water prior to consumption to prevent this material from getting into the body. Such procedures, however, should not interfere with tactical operations.

(1) *Food.* All unpackaged and uncovered foods, such as vegetables, fruits, and carcass meats, should be considered contaminated if obtained from a known fallout field or a reading of more than twice background is obtained when the food supplies are monitored with the AN/PDR 27 radiac set with probe window open. Monitoring of the food must be conducted in an area of low background radiation so that greater accuracy can be achieved. Fresh fruits, vegetables, and carcass meats can be decontaminated by washing, trimming, or peeling the outer skin or leaves. Nothing should be thrown away or destroyed. Nonperishable items that cannot be readily decontaminated, such as flour, sugar or salt, can be set aside allowing natural radioactive decay to reduce the radioactivity to acceptable levels. If food supplies are critically low, contaminated food may have to be consumed. In this event, it may be advisable to dilute the contamination by mixing with uncontaminated food. This will reduce the total amount of radioactivity to a level where exposure will be minimal. Boiling or cooking contaminated food has no effect in removing the fallout material.

(a) In packaged containers, such as cans, fiberboard, cellophane, most of the contamination is not in the food but on the package. The simple expedient of brushing, or washing the dust from the container will remove most of the radioactive material.

(b) Food animals, such as cattle, hogs, goats, sheep, and poultry that have been exposed to fallout should be considered fit for consumption and slaughtered using routine procedures. Mild radiation sickness in animals does not necessarily mean that they cannot be used as food. Even if the animals have been exposed to an internal radiation hazard, they can still be used as food as long as the internal organs are discarded during butchering. Chickens that have eaten radioactive material may lay contaminated eggs, but most of the radioactivity will be concentrated in the shells. The white and yolks will be free of significant radiation and can be eaten without harm. It is probable that chickens will not lay if the radioactive body burden is large enough that their eggs are unfit to eat.

(c) In some cases, particularly when small weapons are involved, it is possible that food will be exposed to sufficient neutron flux to produce considerable induced radioactivity in the food without it being destroyed by the blast and heat. The elements that are most prominently involved are sodium, potassium, sulfur, copper, bromine, zinc, and especially phosphorous. Consequently, the foods which must be considered with the greatest caution in an area of induced radiation are dairy products, high salt content foods, dry beans, raisins, and ready-mixed cake and biscuit flours. It is important to remember that the elements listed above have isotopes with short half-lives (*for example* sodium–24, 15 hours; potassium–42, 12 hours and phosphorous–32, 14 days) and, therefore, the activity will decay very rapidly. It should be possible to consume foods containing these isotopes within a week or two. Canned foods should not be segregated on the basis of high readings obtained from unopened containers. Cans, particularly those with "C" enamel, may incur a high level of induced activity (from zinc in the enamel, not from iron in the can). Glass, because of its high salt content, will show very high levels of activity, and clear glass will turn brown in color. Container radioactivity has no bearing on the suitability of food for use. This activity is not transferred to the contents, and in many cases, highly active containers will contain food that is entirely safe. No significant toxic byproducts are formed in any of the exposed food.

(2) *Water.* The ingestion of contaminated water can be avoided if certain precautions are taken. It should be pointed out first that it is not the radiation from the fallout that contaminates the water but the fallout itself. If the fallout particles do not physically enter the water, the water does not become contaminated. Water, therefore, in canteens, tanks, water cans, or other

sealed sources will not be contaminated by fallout and will be safe for drinking. The same is usually true from ground sources, such as wells and spring water. Water in pipelines, covered reservoirs, and other containers will be free from radioactive contamination. Water in streams is more likely to contain less radioactivity than that from lakes and ponds due to dilution. In the first few days after nuclear attack, most of the fallout which is deposited on the surface of still bodies or water, such as lakes and ponds, will settle down through the water and come to rest on the bottom. A very small amount of the radioactive material will go into solution and be distributed throughout the water. Therefore, water drawn from below the surface will contain relatively low concentrations of radioactivity. (Submerge a canteen upside down a few centimeters below the surface of the water and when full rapidly withdraw the canteen.) This procedure should be considered only in the event of an emergency. Such water must be disinfected to kill biological contaminants before drinking. Filtering contaminated water through a 15-centimeter (6 inch) column of loose dirt is another emergency procedure that may be used.

(a) It is most unlikely that a casualty producing dose of radiation will be incurred by the consumption of contaminated water. The controlling factor is whether or not the total area in which the surface water has been contaminated is radiologically safe for people to enter in. *If the area is safe enough to be in, the water should be suitable for drinking for limited periods of time.*

(b) The decontamination of water is the responsibility of the Corps of Engineers. Mildly contaminated water can be treated by standard engineer water purification equipment. Contaminated water with excessive amounts of dissolved radioactive material might have to be treated by a combination of standard methods and distillation or ion exchange. The approval of the potability of water is the responsibility of the Medical Service. Quantitative determination of the actual level of contamination of the water from the engineer water point must be made at a medical laboratory. The order of preference in the selection of sources of water (or fluids) in a known fallout field is as follows:

1. Approved engineer water points.
2. Ground water sources (wells and springs).
3. Public water supplies.
4. Water in water trailers, water cans, tanks, and canteens. Bottled soft drinks, canned juices, and other beverages.

5. Fast moving streams.
6. Deep still water sources (lakes and ponds).

b. *Personnel.* The radiological decontamination of personnel should be accomplished as soon as the situation permits. If there is time and the tactical situation permits, personnel should bathe, using plenty of soap and water, preferably warm. Particular attention should be given to skin creases, hairy parts of the body, and the fingernails. Rewashing is accomplished as indicated by monitoring. After decontamination is adequate, as determined by monitoring, personnel should be issued clean clothing. Personnel decontamination stations or quartermaster shower facilities should be used whenever possible. When personnel are prohibited by the tactical situation from using the normal decontamination procedures, they may use field expedient procedures, to include shaking and brushing of clothing. Personnel should wipe all exposed skin with a damp cloth and remove as much radioactive dust as possible from the hair and from under the fingernails. Personnel should bathe and change clothing when the tactical situation permits. Detailed procedures for handling the contaminated patient are described in chapter 7.

c. *Material.* Medical equipment and facilities are also subjected to contamination. Overall or area decontamination procedures are outlined in TM 3–220.

41. Command Radiation Guidance

a. *Definitions.*

(1) *Command radiation guidance.* Advice of the staff surgeon on the effect and influence of predicted and actual radiation received by a command.

(2) *Operational exposure guidance (OEG).* The maximum amount of nuclear radiation which the commander considers his unit may be permitted to receive while performing a particular mission or missions.

b. *General.* To make proper decisions, a commander needs information on both the present and the future health of his command. On the battlefield, health is affected by trauma and disease. Radiation sickness is a disease. The effect on the present health of a command of a particular disease is merely a tabulation of the daily reports of subordinate units. To predict the effect of a given disease on the future health of a command requires a reliable military experience factor. There is no such factor for radiation sickness. Therefore, to comment intelligently and reliably, the staff surgeon must familiarize himself with the present state of our knowledge and examine the parameters which influence his advice.

c. Parameters.

(1) *Biological effects.* Table 9, lists the acute effects of whole-body irradiation. This dose effect relationship holds for doses received within 1–2 days. The data applies to groups, and effects on individuals may vary considerably from these predictions. Note that individuals receiving 200 rads or more will probably require hospitalization at some time following their exposure. With significant doses, nausea and vomiting occur early, usually within 1–3 hours.

(2) *Physical effectiveness.* Generally, when we speak of an effective individual, we mean one who is capable of carrying out an assigned mission or task. Some tasks require a high degree of physical and/or mental effectiveness; others require a relatively low degree. To illustrate, the degree of physical effectiveness required to perform typical military combat tasks has been estimated to be as follows:

(a) Fire a preplaced weapon_____10%

(b) Operate radio communications_20%

(c) Drive a vehicle_____50%

(d) Aim a weapon_____80%

(e) Assault a position_____90%

(f) Hand-to-hand combat _____90+%

In any attempt, therefore, to relate radiation dose to individual effectiveness, one must consider the task for which effectiveness is being determined. Although individual effectiveness may be of concern, command elements at higher levels are more likely to be interested in effectiveness of units rather than individuals. It has been estimated that 10 to 30 percent ineffectiveness in a unit may render that unit incapable of accomplishing its mission. However, it is not always a matter of how many ineffectives there are in a unit so much as who these casualties are. Loss of the surgeons of a mobile surgical hospital would render the unit completely ineffective so far as accomplishing its primary mission. Predicting the point at which radiation exposure will result in individual or unit ineffectiveness is almost impossible since adequate human data is lacking. The combination of variations in exposure, and biological response makes sudden, simultaneous loss of all personnel in a unit unlikely. Generally, the unit commander and the surgeon should have ample time to evaluate unit effectiveness as individuals become sick.

(3) *Recovery rates.*

(a) One of the more important and uncertain factors which limits our ability to predict personnel effectiveness is that of recovery from radiation injury. There is ample evidence that recovery takes place but the rate and the degree is questionable. There is also reasonable certainty that some residual injury remains after recovery but once again there is insufficient evidence at this time to state how much. Recovery rates now in use are really little more than educated guesses. Recovery rates are variously estimated to be 2.5 percent to 10 percent of the unrecovered portion of the injury per day. The residual irreparable injury is variously considered to be from 0 to 10 percent of the original total exposure.

(b) Little or nothing is known about the effect of successive exposures upon repair which is in progress from a previous radiation injury. There is even some evidence, though inconclusive, that there is a period during recovery when an individual is radio-resistant to new radiation exposures.

(c) Recent experiments with monkeys indicate that partial recovery of effectiveness takes place even at supralethal dose levels (2500–30,000 rads) when received in a very short period of time. This may indicate that heavily irradiated troops may be capable of performing some military tasks during certain periods following exposure. Because of the uncertainty as to recovery and residual injury, it may be advisable to disregard recovery entirely in estimates of troop effectiveness and accept whatever recovery occurs as a bonus or "built-in" safety factor. In general, several conclusions with respect to recovery and the effect of protracted doses can be drawn:

1. Any whole-body gamma dose delivered over a protracted period of time will have a lesser effect than that same dose if delivered in a 24-hour period. Therefore, lives and morbidity can be saved by spreading out radiation exposures in time and among different groups of people when the tactical situation permits.

2. Recovery from radiation injury is probably never complete.

3. Recovery from high level exposures is slower than from low.

4. Partial recovery of effectiveness takes place even at supralethal dose levels.

(4) *Radiation history.* A record of radiation exposure should be kept up to date and available for all units. However, until there is a satisfactory individual dosimeter, individual and unit doses can only be estimated from a few instruments distributed over the unit area. Though the medical officer managing a patient may consider the dose data thus recorded, he must still make his decisions on the basis of the clinical picture presented. Staff surgeons may use dose estimation for units to distinguish exposed from unexposed units

and the various degrees of exposure. A 20 percent higher average reading of one unit's dosimeters over those of another indicates a significant exposure difference. When rapid turnover of military units or personnel occurs, recording and transmitting estimated unit and individual radiation histories will be extremely difficult and subject to many errors.

(5) *Instruments.* In the absence of a biological indicator of absorbed dose, the medical officer is forced to rely on the physical measurement of exposure dose with available instruments. To date, there is no instrument in the field which measures both the prompt gamma and neutron radiation. Gamma measuring field instruments often have an inherent error of ± 20 percent. The surgeon attempting to correlate an instrument reading with biological effects must be aware of the many variables and errors which are present.

d. *Radiation Guidance.*

(1) *Command radiation guidance.*

(a) In lieu of more experience, better instrumentation and a better means to collect and record data, any radiation advice given to the commander must be based not on generalities but on examination of each situation. Table 17 is a simplified dose-effect guideline. Utilizing this table and modifying it with personal experience, the surgeon can give applicable advice.

(b) Situations.

1. With prompt radiation exposure, the surgeon's radiation advice will of necessity be after the fact. In most situations an immediate casualty and damage assessment will determine unit effectiveness. In the few situations where radiation exposure knowledge may be of decisional importance, the biological response time will be shorter than the collecting and recording time of estimated individual doses which are of dubious value in the first place. By evaluating the number of radiation casualties, the onset, type and degree

of symptoms, the surgeon can offer the most meaningful guidance possible.

2. Unlike the situation of exposure to prompt radiation, the commander operating in or through fallout has a greater measure of control over the radiation exposure to his troops. Against his operational choices will be tabulated a series of predicted exposure doses. The surgeon will be asked to comment on each of these. If the unit has no exposure, the surgeon should comment according to paragraph A of table 17. He can emphasize that at 200 rads the commander will pay a severe casualty price for an objective; and at 800 rads a severe mortality price. The present state of our knowledge does not allow an accurate prediction of the percent effected and onset and degrees of effectiveness.

3. For contemplated exposure of a unit in which individuals have varying estimated exposure histories, the surgeon should use paragraph B of table 17. The strength of his advice must, however, lie on medical evaluation. He will know his unit. He can give a general impression of the unit's ability to perform a particular mission by observing the past and present performance, observing the rate of sick call and observing the type and number of symptoms. As with any disease, the surgeon alerts the commander to the deteriorating health status of his command.

(c) The commander is always advised to keep the exposure as low as possible, consistent with the mission. He can know that not all his soldiers will deteriorate to the same degree simultaneously. When possible, the commander should employ units with the least exposure history and longest time since last exposure. As the clinician treats and evacuates soldiers on the basis of symptoms, the staff surgeon can best advise and consent on the basis of symptoms.

(2) *Operation exposure guidance.* Operation exposure guide is a command dose based on overall staff advice. It will vary from situation to situation and most often will be influenced by the mission. Each operations order should have a specified operation exposure guide. It is the maximum amount of nuclear radiation which the commander considers his troops should receive while performing a specific mission. The present Operation Exposure Guide for the U. S. Army is based on Annex E to NATO STANAG (Standardization Agreement) 2083 and is seen in table 18. This operation exposure guide is well within the present knowledge of medical effects. A detailed discussion of the degree of risk categories, radiation

Table 17. Simplified Dose-Effect Relationship

A. *ACUTE DOSE RECEIVED WITHIN 24–48 HOURS*

25 RADS	Blood effects threshold.
100 RADS	Symptom threshold.
200 RADS	Casualty threshold.
400 RADS	50% mortality.
800 RADS	Approaching 100% mortality.

B. *CHRONIC DOSES LIKELY TO PRODUCE CASUALTIES*

200 RADS	in a week.
300 RADS	in a month.
500 RADS	in a year.

Table 18. Operation Exposure Guide

Radiation status [2, 5]	Total past cumulative dose [4]	Single exposure criteria [1, 3]	
RS–1 Units	<75 rad	Negligible Risk	≦5 rad
		Moderate Risk	>5 rad≦20 rad
		Emergency Risk	>20 rad≦50 rad
RS–2 Units	75–150 rad	All further exposure considered Moderate or Emergency Risk.	
		Moderate Risk	≦5 rad
		Emergency Risk	>5 rad≦20 rad
RS–3 Units	>150 rad (Threshold for onset of combat ineffectiveness)	All further exposure considered Emergency Risk.	
		Emergency Risk	<5 rad

NOTES

[1] For operations in radiologically contaminated areas, the operation exposure guide established by the commander can be any number in the risk range appropriate to the unit's mission and radiation status.

[2] Radiation status categories are based on previous exposure to radiation.

[3] Risk levels are graduated within each status category in order to provide more stringent criteria as the total radiation dose accumulated becomes more serious.

[4] All exposures to radiation are considered to be total body and simply additive. No allowance is made for body recovery from radiation injury.

[5] Reclassification of units from a more serious radiation status category, to a less serious one, is done by the commander upon advice of the surgeon after ample observation of actual state of health of the exposed personnel has been made.

data processing, and the role of the surgeon is contained in chapter VII, FM 3–12.

42. Casualty Estimation

a. Although it is not a designated responsibility of the surgeon to estimate the approximate casualty load and types of casualties following a nuclear attack upon friendly forces, the surgeon of an affected command should make such an appraisal as rapidly as possible to determine the immediate medical support required in the damaged area.

b. The *Handbook for the Estimation of Battle Casualties (Nuclear) 1963* outlines a system for medical service users in the field. This handbook provides a series of tables which are estimates of the kinds of casualties (blast, thermal, nuclear radiation, and combinations) by percent which may be produced by a nuclear detonation. It does not include losses caused by exposure to fallout. Although this system was designed for war games, field exercises and maneuvers, it may be used in lieu of actual experience in planning medical support requirements.

c. Guidance for the medical planner in estimating losses in nuclear warfare is also found in chapter 2, FM 101–10–3.

CHAPTER 10

NUCLEAR WEAPON ACCIDENT HAZARDS

43. General

Extreme care has been devoted to the design of nuclear weapons to prevent a nuclear yield in the event of accidental detonation, and to the development of safe procedures for handling and transporting them. Nevertheless, accidents by their very nature, are completely unpredictable and consideration must be given to all conceivable hazards that might arise in the storage or transportation of nuclear weapons or when actually in the delivery vehicle. These hazards may be due to: a) detonation of the high explosive, b) fissionable material, i.e., uranium and plutonium, c) tritium, which is radioactive, d) fission products in the unlikely event of a partial nuclear yield and, e) beryllium and lead.

44. The High Explosive Hazard

a. Most nuclear weapons contain conventional high explosives in varying amounts up to many hundreds of pounds. In any accident involving a nuclear weapon, such as dropping or exposure to fire, there is a possibility that detonation of the high explosive may occur. This constitutes the *major hazard* in dealing with nuclear accidents. One of the characteristics of TNT is the unpredictability of its response to a given stimulus. Thus, impact or a fire may or may not cause a detonation. If a detonation does occur, it can range from a very small one to one of considerable magnitude or it may be a series of small explosions. The breakup of the weapon due to impact or a small explosion will probably result in local scattering of small pieces of high explosive. These may burn and possibly explode.

b. Rough handling of high explosives as well as accidents can lead to the formation of powdered explosive. Under these conditions, most explosive materials are more unstable than in bulk form and are more apt to be detonated by shock or change in temperature. Exposure to sunlight also increases the sensitivity of high explosives. At the same time there is a change in color which makes small pieces and powder difficult to distinguish from their surroundings. Thus, it is unwise for

anyone other than trained ordnance disposal personnel to attempt clearing an area of broken high explosives.

c. If a nuclear weapon is exposed to the flames from a gasoline or similar fire, arising from the fuel or propellant of the carrying vehicle, the high explosive may ignite, burn and in some cases, detonate. Fires resulting from large quantities of burning high explosives are very difficult to extinguish. At the same time, acrid, suffocating, and toxic gases are produced, and a poisonous residue may remain. If the high explosive is confined, as in an intact weapon, detonation may occur at any time. In addition, high explosives melt at relatively low temperatures; the heat of the fire may thus cause the molten explosive to flow out of the weapon and then resolidify. In this state, the material is extremely sensitive to shock and may detonate if stepped on.

d. In the event of a nuclear weapon becoming involved in a fire, all persons not essential for damage control or recovery operation should withdraw to a distance of a least 457 meters (1,500 feet) to minimize the injury potential of the blast that may result from the detonation of the high explosive.

e. Because of the formation of the noxious fumes produced by the burning explosive and vehicle fuel that may be present, only those individuals properly protected with respiratory equipment should be permitted to remain in the downwind path of a fire or potential detonation. Smoke may be tolerated for a short period of time if necessary in the interest of saving lives.

45. The Plutonium Hazard

a. *Inhalation Exposure.* Since plutonium is primarily an alpha emitter, it is only a hazard when inside the body. With the accidental detonation of the high explosives in a nuclear weapon, plutonium may be dispersed in the form of finely divided particles or fumes which become airborne. As a result, the primary plutonium hazard at the site of a nuclear weapon accident is inhalation with retention of these particles. Most particles inhaled will not be retained and only the smallest will penetrate deep enough into the pulmonary tissue so that they will be retained. What fraction of the inhaled particles will be retained will depend primarily upon the particle size distribution. In a weapons accident, there is a high probability that the aerosol of plutonium produced will be in the form of a fume with very small particles present. Even allowing for absorption of these on larger inert particles in the atmosphere, there will still be a considerable fraction of plutonium in this form. This is unlike the industrial situation wherein plutonium dusts from machining processes are present which do not include such small size particles.

(1) There is a higher proportion of absorption from the lungs into the circulation when plutonium is in the form of a fume. Plutonium dusts on the other hand are absorbed very slowly and very little can get from the lung tissue through the pulmonary lymphatic barrier and into the general circulation.

(2) To determine the extent of inhalation exposure, nasal swipes should be performed on all personnel who may have been exposed to plutonium. If instrument monitoring of the nasal swipes reads 200 disintegrations per minute or more, urinalyses should be performed. The specimens should be collected and forwarded to an appropriate medical laboratory for analysis. A quantitative urinary plutonium determination will indicate the amount of plutonium which has been absorbed.

(3) If an exposure to plutonium aerosols is suspected, treatment with diethylenetriaminepentacetic acid (DTPA) should be begun immediately to enhance plutonium excretion. The recommended dosage is 1 gram given intravenously by slow drip on alternate days three times a week for 3 weeks. If laboratory reports are later found to be negative, therapy can then be halted. If they are positive, treatment should be continued and even repeated if thought necessary. If repeated, renal function must be followed carefully because of the possibility of renal tubular damage from the DTPA.

b. *Skin Contamination.* Skin contamination with plutonium may be detected by monitoring with the gamma probe of the AN/PDR-60 instrument. This is possible because there is a weak gamma photon emitted along with each alpha particle. Washing with soap and water will remove over 65 percent of the plutonium contamination, and washing plus alternate applications of 4 percent $KMnO_4$ and 5 percent $NaHSO_3$ is over 98 percent effective.

c. *Wound Contamination.*
(1) Plutonium introduced into the skin and subcutaneous tissue through lacerations and puncture wounds may remain at the site of the wound for a very long time. Thus, alpha radiation of the surrounding tissue with the associated inflammatory response and intense scarring may produce severe local damage, and loss of function. The probability of the occurrence of a neoplasm is unknown but small tumors have been found. These effects are long term and are not important in combat.

(2) The extent of contamination of lacerations and puncture wounds may be estimated by external measurement with the gamma probe of the AN/PDR-60. However, the gamma rays which are being measured are weak and easily attenuated by tissue. In addition, the diameter of the gamma probe precludes accurate localization of the plutonium particles.

(3) Extensive wound debridement for the purpose of removing plutonium particles is not indicated; only routine wound debridement and thorough surgical cleansing is necessary. When delayed wound closure is being used in combat, daily irrigation prior to the time of closure could be done. This could result in the removal of some superficial particles missed with the first irrigation.

(4) In the case of abrasions, over 50 percent of the plutonium contamination is removed by normal surgical cleansing, and most of the remainder is removed when the scab is sloughed.

d. *Prevention and Control.* Studies to date indicate that the plutonium hazard at the site of a nuclear accident is not great. However, if monitoring instruments indicate a plutonium hazard, protective clothing and respiratory protective devices should be worn. Surfaces must be monitored to determine the magnitude of the contamination. Particle air sampling must be performed to properly evaluate the hazard caused by plutonium air suspensions. Table 19 provides guidance as to protection standards required for personnel.

46. The Uranium Hazard

a. *General.* Uranium is only 1/500 as hazardous as plutonium from the standpoint of radiation. However, the chemical toxicity hazard (acute renal tubular necrosis) of uranium is significant. Inhalation is the primary means of entry. Significant numbers of uranium particles small enough to be retained in the lungs may be expected only over a small area near a nuclear weapons accident site. It is unlikely that alpha radiation levels above 1,000 dpm/m^3 will ever be encountered in an accident. However, the possibility of hazardous airborne contamination must be considered.

Table 19. Short Exposure Respiratory Protection Standards

Exposure level (Alpha disintegration)	Respiratory protection for short term exposure *
0 to 100 dpm/m³	No respiratory protection.
100 to 10,000 dpm/m³	High-filtration respirator at least 99% efficient (such as the M9A1 protective mask).
100 to 100,000 dpm/m³	High-filtration respirator at least 99.9% efficient (such as the ABC–M17 protective mask or the M9A1 protective mask with the M14 biological and radiological particulate canister).
Greater than above levels	Self-contained breathing apparatus.

* Short term exposure is defined as no more than several working days per month.

b. *Management.* The principles outlined for the management of plutonium contaminated patients also apply to casualties exposed to uranium.

47. The Tritium Hazard

a. *General.* Tritium, which is used in nuclear weapons, represents a beta radiation hazard. Tritium oxide or heavy water (T_2O), which is the actual form which presents the hazard, has to be absorbed to be dangerous. Skin and pulmonary absorption occur readily and are equally important as routes of entry. Tritium oxide is also absorbed readily from the gastrointestinal tract but this is a less probable route of entry. Following absorption, tritium oxide is distributed throughout the body just as is water. The beta radiations emitted during tritium decay are very weak (6 Kev), but they produce essentially whole-body radiation injury because of the distribution of heavy water.

b. *Absorption of Tritium.* When a man is exposed to an atmosphere containing tritium oxide, he will absorb through the respiratory tract about 98 to 99 percent of the tritium oxide inspired. This substance may also gain entrance to the body following skin contact with contaminated surfaces. The release of tritium oxide into a closed space (nuclear weapon storage sites, laboratories, or industrial plants) may constitute a very serious hazard. More than a lethal quantity of tritium oxide can be inhaled in one breath of air saturated with tritium oxide vapor. Skin absorption may also occur if tritium oxide contaminated metals found at a nuclear accident site are handled without the use of protective rubber gloves.

c. *Detection of Exposure.* Urine assay for tritium is the only means of measuring the degree of exposure of an individual. It is, therefore, imperative that persons working with tritium oxide or tritium-contaminated materials submit routine urine samples. The frequency of sampling should be determined by the amount of tritium handled and the prevailing working conditions. When tritium oxide exposure is suspected, urine samples should be obtained immediately, at 30 minutes, and at 3-hour intervals thereafter. Followup specimens should be obtained as indicated. Specimens should be forwarded to the United States Army Environmental Hygiene Agency, Edgewood, Maryland, 21040, or other laboratory capable of making this determination. If urinary determinations indicate more than 47 microcuries of tritium per liter, the maximum permissible body burden of tritium (2 millicuries) has been exceeded, and treatment should be instituted.

d. *Therapy.* A high oral fluid intake should be administered following tritium exposure. Unless contraindicated from a cardiovascular-renal standpoint, several liters of fluid should be ingested during the first 24 hours following exposure. Diuretic drugs may also be used to enhance urinary excretion of tritium oxide. On a normal fluid intake, one-half of the tritium oxide will be eliminated from the body in about 12 days. By administering a high fluid intake, the half-time for elimination can be reduced to 2 days.

e. *Prevention.* Prevention of tritium exposure includes the use of monitoring instruments, protective plastic clothing, rubber gloves, and respiratory protective devices.

(1) Tritium monitoring instruments do not differentiate between tritium gas and tritium oxide vapor. Therefore, it is always necessary to assume that tritium oxide vapor is present if an exposure has occurred.

(2) Self-contained breathing apparatus and impermeable clothing (e.g., polyvinyl chloride suits) should be used by personnel working in tritium-contaminated areas. However, significant amounts of tritium oxide may penetrate even plastic suits if they are exposed to high concentrations. Exposures of personnel using the suits can be controlled by establishing working time limits based on the expected penetration. Laundering does not appear to affect overall permeability of polyvinyl chloride clothing.

(3) Since tritium oxide vapor passes through the rubber in hours or less, rubber gloves should be changed frequently. Tritium-contaminated materials should always be handled with rubber gloves to prevent skin absorption of tritium oxide.

(4) Tritium-contaminated surfaces should

be washed with water and a detergent or organic solvents.

(5) The tritium inhalation exposure hazard at the site of a nuclear accident should be negligible. The main consideration is the prevention of skin absorption of tritium by requiring personnel to wear rubber gloves when handling tritium-contaminated metal fragments.

48. Other Possible Hazards

a. Beryllium and Lead. Beryllium and lead may also be used in nuclear weapons and may represent health hazards if fire or explosion occurs. Beryllium inhaled in the form of fumes, dusts, or smokes may result in a pulmonary granulomatosis. Contamination of wounds can occur and may result in delayed wound healing and the formation of chronic ulcers. Rubber gloves should be worn when beryllium compounds are handled, and protective respiratory devices should be used in beryllium-contaminated areas. Lead poisoning may occur following the inhalation of fumes or smokes, but appropriate respiratory devices will protect against this hazard.

b. Fission Products. These elements would not be found at a nuclear accident site unless the explosion involved at least a partial nuclear yield. This possibility is extremely remote and has not been observed in any of the nuclear weapons accidents to date. Calculations indicate that an explosion of a few pounds of TNT would result in significant local nuclear radiation contamination. Therefore, beta-gamma monitoring should always be performed at the site of a nuclear weapons accident. If gamma radiation is detected, and the presence of fission products from a partial yield would be likely the procedures and principles outlined in chapter 9 should be followed.

49. Radiological Emergency Medical Teams

In the event of a nuclear accident occurring in CONUS, Radiological Emergency Medical Teams (REMT) have been organized, trained, and equipped to be deployed at a nuclear accident site. The REMT is composed of a team leader (Medical Corps Officer) and at least three other qualified individuals. Its functions are—

   a. Monitoring casualties for radiological health hazards and exposure level criteria.

   b. Evaluating prevailing survey data to provide guidance to the responsible army area representative regarding the release of contaminated areas.

   c. Monitoring medical facilities and equipment where contaminated patients have been evacuated.

   d. Advising on containment of radiological hazards and decontamination of exposed patients, medical personnel, medical facilities and equipment.

   e. Advising on pertinent early and followup laboratory and clinical procedures.

In addition to the above, the REMT personnel are prepared to assist with essential emergency medical care.

APPENDIX A

REFERENCES

	AR 40-5	Preventive Medicine
	AR 40-14	Control and Recording Procedures: Occupational Exposure to Ionizing Radiation
	AR 220-58	Organization and Training for Chemical, Biological and Radiological Operations
	AR 320-5	Dictionary of United States Army Terms
	AR 385-30	Safety Color Code Markings and Signs
	FM 3-10	Employment of Biological Agents
	FM 3-12	Operational Aspects of Radiological Defense
	FM 3-15	Nuclear Accident Contamination Control
	FM 5-15	Field Fortifications
	FM 8-10	Medical Service Theater of Operations
	FM 8-55	Army Medical Service Planning Guide
	FM 21-10	Military Sanitation
	FM 21-40	Chemical, Biological and Nuclear Defense
	FM 21-41	Soldiers Handbook for Chemical and Biological Operations and Nuclear Warfare
	FM 101-10 (part I)	Staff Officers Field Manual Organization, Technical, and Logistical Data
(S)	FM 101-10-3	Staff Officers Field Manual Organizational, Technical, and Logistical Data, Classified Data (U)
	FM 101-31-1	Staff Officers Field Manual: Nuclear Weapons Employment
	TC 3-15	Prediction of Fallout from Atomic Demolition Munitions (ADM)
	TM 3-210	Fallout Prediction
	TM 3-220	Chemical, Biological, and Radiological (CBR) Decontamination
	TM 3-240	Field Behavior of Chemical, Biological and Radiological Agents
	TM 5-311	Military Protective Construction (Nuclear Warfare and Chemical and Biological Operations)
	TM 10-277	Protective Clothing for Chemical Operations
(C)	TM 23-200	Capabilities of Nuclear Weapons (U)
	TB Med 246	Medical Management of Mass Casualties in Nuclear Warfare
	DA Pam 39-3	Nuclear Weapons
	DA Pam 108-1	Index of Army Films, Transparencies, GTA, Charts and Recordings
(S)	USACDCNG 62-8	Criteria for Nuclear Weapon Personnel Safety and Casualties (U)

"Handbook for the Estimation of Battle Casualties (Nuclear)," WRAIR, WRAMC, Washington, D. C. 20012

NBS Handbook 59, Permissible Dose from External Sources of Ionizing Radiation

NATO Handbook, "Emergency War Surgery," 1958; U. S. Government Printing Office, Washington, D. C.

"Symposium on the Management of Mass Casualties," Medical Field Service School, Brooke Army Medical Center, Ft Sam Houston, Texas, 1964

"Biological and Environmental Effects of Nuclear Warfare," Hearing before Special Subcommittee on Radiation, Joint Committee on Atomic Energy, Congress of the U. S., 86th Congress, June 22-26, 1959, Washington, D. C., U. S. Government Printing Office, 1959

MF 8–7897	The Medical Effects of Nuclear Radiation
MF 20–7815	The Effects of Atomic Bomb Explosions
MF 20–8148	Radioactive Contamination
MF 20–9311	Atomic Weapons and Fire
TF 3–2499	Individual Protection against CBR Attack
TF 3–2602	This is Atomic, Biological and Chemical Warfare
TF 8–2881	Medical Effects of Nuclear Weapons
TF 8–3143	Radioactive Contamination of Food and Water
TF 8–2675	Management of Mass Casualties—Sorting
TF 8–2676	Management of Mass Casualties—Wounds
TF 8–2712	Management of Mass Casualties—Psychological Casualties
TF 8–2713	Management of Mass Casualties—Burns
TF 11–2234	Fundamentals of Radiac Instruments
TF 11–2531	Individual Protection Against Atomic Attack

AN EXAMPLE OF AN SOP FOR HANDLING RADIOACTIVELY CONTAMINATED PATIENTS IN A FIELD HOSPITAL

I. PURPOSE

The purpose of this SOP is to establish procedures designed to protect the patients and medical personnel in the field hospital from the harmful effects of fallout contamination.

II. APPLICATION

This SOP will be executed upon receipt of notification that the hospital is receiving patients who are contaminated with fallout but the hospital itself is not in a contaminated area.

III. CAUTION

These Standing Operating Procedures deal with a minor hazard. The radiological contamination of patients will not interfere with the best possible medical care of these patients.

IV. PROCEDURES

A. All Personnel.

All personnel except those who are assigned duties by this SOP will continue their normal duties. The provisions of the SOP will insure adequate protection to the patients and all medical personnel.

B. Radiac Monitors.

1. Number of monitors—2
2. Special clothing—None.
3. Equipment: AN/PDR–27, c/w case (2 each).
4. Report to: Receiving Station.
5. Duties:

a. Check the AN/PDR–27 for correct functioning in accordance with the operator's instruction manual. If it is not functioning properly, replace the batteries as indicated.

b. Measure the background radiation with the beta shield removed from the probe. All incoming patients will be considered contaminated if reading is twice current background or higher.

c. Inform hospital commander or CBR officer of the arrival of contaminated patients.

d. Monitor all incoming patients using headset. Scan patient with unshielded probe at 15 centimeters (6 inches) from patient's body. Pay particular attention to the shoes. If the reading is twice background or greater, write "Radiological Contamination" (RADCON) on the patient's EMT.

e. Twice daily one monitor will go through the hospital and check each contaminated patient. If a patient is free from contamination, his EMT will be marked "Decontaminated—date and hour" beside the phrase "Radiological Contamination" (RADCON). If a patient is not free from contamination, the nurse in charge will be informed.

f. The monitor who is dispatched through the hospital will monitor litters and other items which have been decontaminated and will release those items found to be uncontaminated. Those items which have not been adequately decontaminated will be returned to the persons who have responsibility for their decontamination.

C. Responsibilities of Persons in Charge of Wards.

1. All incoming contaminated patients will be bathed as soon as practicable. Particular attention should be paid to the parts of the body which are normally exposed. The patient's hair will be monitored after the rest of the head and neck have been washed. If the scalp is contaminated, the hair will be clipped and the scalp will be washed.

2. The patient's clothes, washcloth, towel, and linens used during the decontamination will be placed in a specially designated hamper. The hamper need not be removed immediately from the ward area. However, there is a hazard from the hamper and extensive pileup of contaminated material must not occur. All personnel who handle contaminated patients or equipment will wear gloves.

3. Contaminated Litters:

a. If the patient is to remain on the litter, brush off dust or mud and wipe handles with damp washcloth.

b. After a patient is removed from a litter, set it aside. It should be washed by the personnel who customarily wash soiled litters. After it has been monitored by the radiac monitor and found to be effectively decontaminated, it should be returned to general use.

4. Contaminated patients need not be isolated from other patients either before or after bathing.

5. Questions concerning contamination should be directed to the CBR officer.

D. Contaminated Clothes Handlers.

1. A detail from supply will collect contaminated clothing on the wards at regular intervals.

2. Contaminated clothing will be kept in a separate container.

3. The disposition of clothing will depend on Quartermaster plans for support of the hospital but in general the following paragraph will apply unless contrary orders are issued:

a. Serviceable clothing will be turned in to the Quartermaster Laundry identified as radioactively contaminated clothing.

b. Serviceable boots will be returned to patients: Discard shoelaces, scrub exterior surfaces with scrub brush and hot soapy water without needlessly wetting the inside of the boot. Radiac monitors will check boots before reissue.

c. Unserviceable clothing and boots will be turned into the QM Salvage Collecting Point identified as radioactively contaminated items.

4. Unnecessary occupancy of areas within 1.8 meter (6 feet) of filled bags of contaminated clothing or boots will be avoided.

COMMAND LINE

OFFICIAL:
(Signed by S3)

APPENDIX C

AN EXAMPLE OF A FALLOUT SOP FOR A MEDICAL UNIT

ANNEX G (PROTECTION AGAINST RADIOLOGICAL FALLOUT)—(WITH 6 APPENDIXES) TO 9TH EVACUATION HOSPITAL FIELD SOP

_____(DATE)

I. GENERAL

A. Purpose. To provide for the protection of unit personnel and patients against fallout radiation.

B. Application.

1. This SOP applies to all personnel, sections, and patients of this hospital. Specific exceptions will be made by the Hospital Commander only.

2. This SOP will become effective whenever nuclear warfare has commenced or is considered likely, or upon direction of the Hospital Commander.

C. Organization. No change except—

a. A Radiological Operations Center (ROC) for the hospital will be established as a part of the hospital headquarters as provided herein.

b. A CBR officer, an Assistant CBR officer, and a CBR NCO will be designated. These will be additional duties.

c. At least one Monitor and Survey Team (M & S Team) of two men will be organized for *each* authorized monitoring or surveying radiac instrument. M & S Team assignments are additional duties.

D. Duties and Responsibilities.

1. Executive officer. Disseminate the warnings "Prepare for Fallout" or "Fallout" as prescribed in this SOP.

2. CBR officer.

a. Provide technical advice and assistance to the Hospital Commander.

b. Establish and operate the ROC when required.

c. Process radiological intelligence received, reported, and generated, including to and from higher and adjacent headquarters.

d. Inspect radiac equipment to insure its readiness at all times.

e. Secure all possible information concerning nuclear detonations, fallout patterns, and radiation intensities relative to any fallout affecting or expected to affect this unit.

f. Supervise construction of and/or assure adequacy of all trenches, foxholes, basements and sandbagging, designed to provide protection against fallout radiation.

g. Direct and supervise monitoring and surveying operations.

h. Supervise and make recommendations concerning conduct of all types of radiological decontamination.

i. Inspect unit radiac equipment and assure its readiness at all times.

j. In conjunction with the training officer, supervise and assure the adequacy of radiological defense training of all unit personnel, including their readiness to implement this SOP. Supervise and assure the adequacy of training of monitors and surveyors, Assistant CBR Officer, and CBR NCO.

k. Assist the Hospital Commander in site organization for ease of fallout protection.

l. Move to new site with advance party to initiate planning and construction or preparation of fallout shelter.

3. Supply officer.

a. Maintain in readiness for instant use, decontamination and radiological defense equipment such as shovels, sandbags, water hoses, batteries for radiac instruments, in such quantities as are determined necessary by the CBR officer.

b. Carry out decontamination operations under supervision of the CBR officer. (Personnel for details to be furnished by the Detachment Commander.)

c. Upon warning "Prepare for Fallout" or notification of "Fallout," see that water distribution is made in accordance with this SOP.

4. Mess officer. Procure sufficient C-type or other packaged rations for unit personnel plus patients, and upon warning "Prepare for Fallout" or notification of "Fallout," make distribution of rations in accordance with this SOP.

5. Assistant CBR officer.

a. Assist the CBR officer.

b. Assume the duties of the CBR officer in his absence.

6. Detachment commander.

a. Provide personnel details to the Supply officer and CBR officer as required.

b. At the command "Prepare for Fallout" or "Fallout," assist the mess officer in distributing rations to detachment EM (may be delegated to the First Sergeant).

7. CBR NCO.

a. Direct monitor and survey activities.

b. Assist the CBR officer.

8. CBR Monitor and Survey Teams. See appendix 5.

E. Reports.

1. The ROC will report the following to higher headquarters.

a. Time of arrival of fallout (1 rad/hr and rising).

b. When unshielded dose rate drops to 1 rad/hr.

c. When unit is forced to consume radiologically contaminated water. (See app 4.)

2. ROC will keep Hospital Commander informed of the radiological situation at all times.

II. COORDINATION OF TACTICAL OPERATIONS.

A. Training.

1. Radiological defense training for all unit personnel will be scheduled and supervised by the S–3 in coordination with the CBR officer. The CBR officer will supervise specialized or technical radiological defense training.

2. A rehearsal of the operations portion of this SOP will be conducted at least yearly, and whenever major changes are made in the SOP.

B. Operations.

1. General.

a. Whenever nuclear warfare has started, is considered likely, or upon order of the Hospital Commander:

(1) A radiation background reading will be made in the open with a radiac rate meter hourly on the hour.

(2) Two IM–93 tactical dosimeters will be located outside Hospital Headquarters tent in an unsheltered location 91 centimeters (3 feet) above the ground. Readings will be taken twice daily at 1000 and 1600 hours. Dosimeters will be recharged at least weekly and will be protected from direct contamination.

(3) A background radiation reading of twice normal or any definite dose reading on the IM–93s will be reported to the CBR officer at once.

b. Shelter.

(1) Whenever possible, the hospital will be located to take advantage of existing fallout shelter (basements, tunnels, caves, field fortifications and stone buildings).

(2) The hospital will not necessarily occupy fallout shelter in normal (nonfallout) operation, whether shelter is existing or field expedient. However, all personnel must be prepared to move into shelter upon implementation of this SOP.

(3) The advance party will commence cleanup and improvement of existing shelter at the new site prior to occupation by the main body. For this reason, the CBR officer will accompany the advance party to the new site, leaving his assistant and/or the CBR NCO at the main hospital site.

(4) Unless adequate existing shelter is available, prior to sleeping in a new site, unit personnel will dig two-man foxholes no less than 46 centimeters (18 inches) deep and large enough to lie in. Pup tents will be erected over these foxholes. This aplies to the advance party as well as the main hospital unit. At the discretion of the Hospital Commander (or Advance Party Commander), other unit personnel may prepare holes for certain designated personnel whose full attention is required for other duties.

(5) Two-man foxholes will be prepared at each guard post and at the hospital ambulance entrance.

(6) As time permits, all shelters (including foxholes, trenches, and existing shelter) will be improved by deepening, undercutting, covering, sandbagging, and any other measures designed to improve the comfort and/or protection of the shelter.

(7) See appendix 2 for measures to be taken when the hospital cannot be accommodated in existing shelter.

2. Action prior to fallout.

a. Warning. The order "Prepare for Fallout" will be disseminated by the Executive officer throughout the hospital area by telephone and/or voice when—

(1) A nuclear burst is observed from the hospital area.

(2) A warning of possible fallout is received from an authorized source.

(3) Ordered by the Hospital Commander.

b. Upon receipt of the order "Prepare for Fallout":

(1) The CBR officer will establish the Radiological Operations Center (ROC) with as-

sistance of members of Headquarters Section and CBR personnel (app. 3).

(2) Chiefs of Services will order ward personnel to (if assistance is required, details will be requested from the Detachment Commander)—

(a) Prepare patients for movement to shelter.

(b) Direct ambulatory patients to shelter. Ambulatory patients who are able will carry litter patients.

(c) Move essential supplies and equipment for patient care to designated shelter areas. A minimum of two blankets, a sleeping bag or an evacuation bag will accompany each patient to shelter.

(3) Mess officer—Deliver three days rations to—

(a) Trenches, basements, or other shelters comprising the patient shelter area.

(b) The Hospital Headquarters.

(c) Each unit EM and each unit officer not occupying patients' shelter or HQ shelter. Pickup will be accomplished at the mess tent with assistance of the First Sergeant in roster checkoff.

(4) Supply officer.

(a) Move water trailers or vehicles to a location accessible to patient shelters with a minimum of radiation exposure of occupants.

(b) Deliver filled 5-gallon cans of water to the EM shelter area (minimum of 20 cans to be distributed by the First Sergeant) and to Hospital Headquarters (minimum of two cans).

(c) Place unexposed X-ray film in a hole in the floor or a niche dug into the side of patient shelter. (Hole should be at least 91 centimeters (3 feet) deep and covered with two layers of sandbags or the equivalent in loose earth.)

(5) Monitoring and Surveying Teams.

(a) Report to CBR officer in Hospital Headquarters.

(b) Check all equipment.

(6) All personnel.

(a) Fill canteens and wear them.

(b) Attach entrenching tools to web belt.

(c) Report to place of duty for instructions.

3. Action during fallout.

a. If fallout commences without prior warning, all actions indicated in paragraph B2 above will be accomplished without delay.

b. Fallout warning.

(1) When unshielded dose rate of 1 rad/hr is read anywhere in the hospital area, it will be reported to the CBR officer.

(2) CBR officer will report same to Hospital Commander.

(3) Upon order of the Hospital Commander, the Executive Officer will spread the command "Fallout" throughout the hospital area by all available means.

c. The Executive Officer will notify next higher headquarters of the onset of fallout by the most expeditious means. Request will be made for the diversion of patients from this hospital, including those already en route, if possible.

d. Personnel not already in shelter will move to shelter.

(1) Movement of patients to shelter will be completed as quickly as possible.

(2) Professional personnel (both doctors and nurses) will enter patient shelter area with the patients and disperse in the shelters according to instructions of their respective Chiefs of Services.

(3) EM not retained by their respective officers or NCOs for duty elsewhere will go to their foxholes in the unit bivouac area.

(4) Designated personnel will enter eight-man shelter in Hospital Headquarters.

(5) Guards will enter perimeter foxholes in pairs.

(6) Two guards for traffic direction will enter foxholes at hospital ambulance entrance.

(7) Other officer personnel without specific tasks or allocated shelters will enter the patient shelter system.

(8) All personnel will take bed roll and/or a minimum of two blankets plus a shelter half or poncho to shelters with them.

(9) Personnel authorized a weapon will take weapon and two clips of ammunition to shelter.

e. Departure from shelter during fallout.

(1) All personnel will remain in shelter until released by order of the Hospital CO unless specifically authorized to leave shelter sooner to perform a specific task.

(2) Permission to leave shelter can only be granted by the Hospital Commander or officers or NCOs specifically designated by him. Time limits will be included in each such clearance.

(3) Prior to authorized departure from shelter, the departing individual will be briefed by a monitor on precautions to be observed. The monitor will clip an IM–93 to the departee's clothing. When the individual returns, the same monitor will see that he brushes himself off, will read his exposure, and report it to the ROC.

(4) All reasonable measures will be taken to prevent excessive radiation exposure of

any individual or group. These measures will include rotation of personnel who leave shelter.

f. Personnel (including able patients) who are in open holes or under tentage will work continuously from the time fallout starts until after the peak intensity is passed, to reduce the direct radiation dose during this period.

(1) Designated personnel under tentage will beat the underside of the tent roof vigorously and frequently to cause fallout material to slide from the roof.

(2) Personnel in open holes or trenches will scrape the bottom of the hole thoroughly and throw scrapings well over the side.

g. As soon as the peak is passed (dose rates are dropping) and notification is spread throughout the hospital, as provided in paragraph 5b(9(b), appendix 3, personnel in open holes or under tentage will—

(1) Make a last good cleanup of fallout material. Repeat and complete all actions listed in paragraph f above.

(2) If flies have been placed over tent roofs, designate personnel to remove the flies quickly in such a manner as to remove most of the fallout material with them. Individuals will then return to shelter immediately.

h. Personnel, including able patients, will continue to improve the protection of shelter.

(1) Side walls of trenches and foxholes can be undercut to afford greater overhead protection.

(2) Overhead covers supporting several inches of earth may be improvised.

(3) All types of holes may be deepened, and if there is sufficient room, deeper holes may be dug in the floor of trenches or other shelters.

(4) Windows and doors of existing shelter may be sandbagged or dirt may be spread over floors above basements to reduce scattered radiation.

i. Redistribution of personnel:

(1) When uniformity of shelter protection has been determined (para 5b(5), app. 3), personnel and patients will be redistributed to achieve maximum radiation protection.

(2) Redistribution within any shelter will be directed by the senior officer present in that shelter.

(3) Redistribution between shelters, if any, will be directed by the Hospital Commander.

4. After fallout.

a. The period after fallout is defined as that period beginning with the resumption of *regular* shifts of work outside shelter, no matter how short the work periods, or the complete

abandoment of shelter, whichever is earlier. The period beginning with the onset of fallout and ending at this point will be referred to as the "acute" phase.

b. The order to resume operation outside shelters normally will not be given prior to the time dose rates have dropped to 1 rad/hr unless ordered by higher headquarters.

c. Evacuation of the site. The unit will evacuate the area and move to a new site under the following conditions:

(1) When ordered to do so by a higher headquarters.

(2) When information available indicates that unit personnel and patients can move to a location of lesser radiation intensity and the dose received during evacuation would be less than that accumulated during continued occupation of the current site. In this case, permission to move must be requested from higher headquarters and approval obtained.

d. The CBR officer will order a survey of the hospital area. Results will be recorded on a rough sketch map and reported to the Commanding Officer. "Hot spots" will be marked and avoided.

e. Decontamination of personnel and patients.

(1) Personnel will practice the best possible personal hygiene during the "acute" phase of fallout and the period immediately following.

(a) Clothing will be brushed or shaken free of dust or mud as often as advised by monitors.

(b) Exposed skin surfaces will be brushed or wiped clean from time to time.

(c) Disabled patients will be cleaned in the same manner.

(2) Containerized (uncontaminated) water will NOT be used for washing or decontamination.

(3) If unit moves to an uncontaminated area or local background drops below 250 mrad/hr—

(a) Monitoring of personnel can be a part of their normal cleanup if time and the situation permit.

(b) An individual may be considered contaminated if an AN/PDR–27 monitoring instrument indicates twice background when probe with open end window is passed approximately 15 centimeters (6 inches) from the body surface.

C. Command and Signal.

1. Command post. Radiological Operations Center in Hospital Headquarters.

2. Liaison will be maintained with—

a. Adjacent military units.

b. The nearest CBROC (whenever possible).

3. Communications.

a. Telephonic communication between hospital headquarters and principal shelter area, including patient shelter area, will be maintained. Shelter areas not in the telephone system will be close enough to a shelter which is in the system to allow voice communication.

b. Noise will be kept to a minimum throughout the hospital area to facilitate voice communication. If available, a PA system with microphone in the ROC will be set up to cover the hospital area.

c. Runners will be employed for communication only when the urgency of the message is commensurate with the exposure to be incurred by the runner in delivering the message.

III. COORDINATION OF ADMINISTRATIVE SUPPORT OPERATIONS

A. *Logistics.*

1. Radiac Instruments—see appendix 6.

2. Food and Water—see appendix 4.

a. Food.

(1) Distribution of packaged rations. Upon command "Prepare for Fallout" or "Fallout," whichever is given earlier, the Mess officer will distribute C-type or other packaged rations as follows:

(a) Three days rations for all anticipated occupants will be delivered to the trenches, basements, or other shelter comprising the patient shelter area.

(b) Three days rations for Hospital Headquarters and ROC personnel will be delivered to the Hospital Headquarters.

(c) Three days rations will be handed to each unit EM or officer not occupying the patient's shelter system or Headquarters shelter. This issue will be made at the mess tent with the assistance of the First Sergeant, who will check off EM by roster.

(2) Subsequent ration issues—see appendix 4.

b. Water.

(1) Upon command "Prepare for Fallout" or "Fallout," whichever is given earlier, the supply officer will—

(a) Move water trailers or vehicles to a location where they are accessible to occupants of patient shelters with a minimum of radiation exposure.

(b) Deliver filled 5-gallon cans of water to the EM bivouac area (minimum of 20 cans to be distributed by the First Sergeant) and to Hospital Headquarters (minimum of two cans).

(2) Upon command "Prepare for Fallout" or "Fallout," whichever is earlier, unit personnel will fill canteens and wear them to shelter.

(3) Containerized (Uncontaminated) water will NOT be used for washing or decontamination.

3. Decontamination.

a. Decontamination materials and equipment will be requisitioned, stored, and issued by the Supply officer in coordination with the CBR officer.

b. The CBR officer will recommend when, where, what, and how decontamination of areas, equipment, building, and supplies will be accomplished.

c. Decontamination operations will be performed under the supervision of qualified monitors.

4. Hospitalization and evacuation.

a. Casualties arriving at the hospital during the "acute" phase of fallout, while personnel are in shelter, will be directed to the patient shelter area by the guard at the hospital ambulance entrance.

b. One entrance to trenches or other shelters in the patient shelter area will be designated for reception of casualties arriving during fallout. This entrance will be clearly marked so that it can be recognized from the ambulance access road.

c. Normal evacuation of patients will be resumed as early as the radiological situation permits.

d. Treatment.

(1) During fallout, patient care and treatment will be continued so far as possible in the same manner and at the same standards as in normal hospital function, *providing* this does not necessitate undue exposure of personnel to radiation.

(2) When personnel and patients are occupying trenches, foxholes, or other field expedient shelter during the "acute" phase of fallout, surgery and treatment will usually be limited to that necessary to save life and limb.

(3) Any individual who exhibits valid symptoms of radiation sickness will be medically evaluated and treated for radiation sickness regardless of the recorded or estimated dose he received.

5. Sanitation. While occupying trenches or foxholes, sanitation and waste disposal will be accomplished through field expedients (such as cat holes and slit trenches). The senior officer or

NCO in each shelter will be responsible for the control of sanitary measures during shelter occupation.

B. Personnel.

1. Subsequent to any period of unit exposure to nuclear radiation, the CBR officer will estimate the average unit exposure, and report same to the Commanding Officer within 12 hours after the completion of the "acute" phase of fallout. Where protection afforded large groups of personnel by different shelters varies significantly, the CBR officer may report two or more average unit exposures, identifying the groups to which each applies.

2. Individual exposures of monitors, survey parties, decontamination crews, late arriving patients, or others who sustained radiation exposures significantly greater than the unit average will be estimated and recorded separately by name in the ROC.

3. Estimated dose to patients will be recorded on each patient's Field Medical Record.

4. Names and estimated doses of each individual will be reported to the Hospital Commander by the CBR officer within 12 hours after the "acute" phase of fallout is over. Negative report will be made.

C. Civil Affairs.

1. Any U. S. or foreign civilians working for the U. S. Army who are present in the unit area at the onset of fallout will be afforded the same protection as military personnel during the "acute" phase.

2. Other civilians will not be taken in for shelter or protection unless there is sufficient food, water, and shelter space to accommodate these civilians without endangering or causing unwarranted discomfort to patients and unit personnel.

COMMAND LINE

APPENDIXES:

1. Appendix 1 (Encountering Fallout While on the Move)

2. Appendix 2 (Fallout Shelter)

3. Appendix 3 (The Radiological Operations Center)

4. Appendix 4 (Food and Water)

5. Appendix 5 (Monitoring and Surveying Teams)

6. Appendix 6 (Radiac Instruments)

OFFICIAL:

(Signed by S3)

APPENDIX 1. ENCOUNTERING FALLOUT WHILE ON THE MOVE (TO ANNEX G TO 9TH EVACUATION HOSPITAL FIELD SOP (app. C))

1. APPLICATION

Provisions of this annex apply to all or any portion of the unit while performing movement other than local movement in the vicinity of an installation.

2. PRIOR TO MARCH

a. Route of march will be reconnoitered if possible. Recon party will note on map all possible fallout shelter enroute.

b. If route reconnaissance is not possible, a map route reconnaissance will be made to determine probable shelter locations along the route of march.

3. DURING THE MARCH

a. As a minimum, the lead vehicle in the column or in each serial of the column will carry a monitor with radiac survey meter, IM–174A. (If available, he may also carry an AN/PDR–27 monitoring instrument.)

b. The lead vehicle in the column or in each serial of the column will also carry one man with a reconnaissance map. He will have indicated on the map the location of all fallout shelter previously determined. At all times he will know the nearest actual shelter already passed and the nearest map-indicated shelter ahead of the column (serial).

c. Intermittent monitoring will be conducted both enroute and at halts (reading at least every 10 minutes).

d. *Continuous monitoring will be ordered when—*

(1) Detonation of a nuclear weapon is observed.

(2) Detonation of a nuclear weapon within 160 kilometers (100 miles) is reported.

(3) Fallout prediction involving route of march is received.

(4) Any IM–174A survey instrument in the column registers visible needle deflection or any reading is obtained on the top (0–500 mrad/hr) scale of an AN/PRD–27 radiac instrument.

(5) Ordered by the convoy or serial commander.

e. *Reports:*

(1) Any monitor initiating continuous monitoring, report same to serial or convoy commander.

(2) Any serial initiating continuous monitoring, report same to convoy commander.

(3) Whenever intensity of 1 rad/hr or higher is encountered, report same to convoy commander.

f. *Action when intensity of 1 rad/hr is encountered.*

(1) Clear the road and halt the column.

(2) Seek shelter.

(a) Limited movement authorized to secure the best shelter available within a reasonable distance.

(b) If no shelter is available, commence preparation of two-man foxholes.

(3) Attempt to secure information concerning the fallout from the nearest CHEMRAD, CBROC, or any unit with whom communication is possible.

(4) At the same time actions in (2) and (3) above are being carried out, attempt to determine whether the field is building up or decaying.

(a) Observe a survey instrument closely (more than one if available) for 15 minutes while the instrument remains in one position and at the same height above the ground. A clear-cut rise in radiation intensity indicates a building-up fallout field. While subsequent action is being taken, continue to observe instruments to confirm or contraindicate build-up of fallout.

(b) Look for ash or dust falling from the sky. Presence indicates a building-up field.

(5) If a clear-cut decision as to whether this is a decaying fallout field or one which is building up cannot be made at this point, send motorized reconnaissance survey party back over the route just covered. Significant radiation intensities in places recently found clear is a positive indication of a building-up fallout field.

(6) *Action when decaying fallout field has been encountered:*

(a) Convoy will pull back to an area of 250 mrad/hr or less.

(*b*) Further attempts will be made to secure information concerning the fallout field.

(*c*) Contact next higher headquarters to report the situation and obtain new orders, if any.

(*d*) Radiological reconnaissance:

1. Reconnoiter to find a route around or through the fallout field with a minimum of exposure to troops.

2. All reconnaissance survey parties will be given intensity, dose, time and/or distance restrictions which they will not exceed. (i.e., return if you encounter intensities exceeding 20 r/hr; do not exceed a dose of 35 rad; do not be gone longer than 1 hour; do not travel more than 24 kilometers (15 miles) from this location—or any combination of limitations.)

3. All reconnaissance parties will carry at least two IM–93 dosimeters in addition to survey meters.

(7) *Action when a building-up fallout field has been encountered:*

(*a*) If local radiation intensities are *increasing rapidly* (more than 2 rad/hr/min on the IM 174A):

1. If possible, report current situation directly or indirectly to next higher headquarters indicating possible delay in carrying out mission.

2. Do not consider evacuation of the fallout area while intensities are rising unless calculation based on reliable information indicates that average dose to unit personnel would be less than 20 r during evacuation. (Sources of reliable information are such agencies as CBROCs, CHEMRADS, S–2 or G–2 or higher staffs, etc.)

3. Initiate intensive action to increase the protection of the shelter presently occupied.

4. During the occupation of shelter, all provisions of paragraph 6, Fallout SOP, will govern just as if the unit were set up in installation.

5. Radiological reconnaissance:

a. Survey reconnaissance parties will NOT be dispatched until ambient intensities begin falling.

b. After radiation intensities begin falling, survey reconnaissance parties may be dispatched only when local dose rate is below 20 rad/hr.

c. First priority for radiological route survey should be in the direction of decreasing radiation intensities, if this can be determined.

d. All survey reconnaissance parties will be given intensity, dose, time, and/or distance restrictions which they will not exceed.

6. Evacuation. Evacuate to a location of 250 mrad/hr or less when reliable information, including survey reconnaissance, indicates that evacuation can be accomplished with less than 20 rad average dose to unit personnel.

7. After evacuation, contact next higher headquarters for orders.

(*b*) If local intensities are relatively static or *increasing slowly* (less than 2 rad/hr/min)—

1. Proceed as in paragraph f(6) above (action when decaying fallout field has been encountered) except—

a. Paragraph (6)(*a*) above. Instead, main body of convoy will remain in shelter and take steps to improve the shelter.

b. In implementation of paragraph (6)(*d*)*2* above, CO will impose more stringent limitations on reconnaissance survey parties in order to provide greater safety factors (i.e., return if you encounter intensities exceeding 15 rad/hr; do not exceed a dose of 25 rad; do not be gone longer than 30 minutes; do not travel further than 16 kilometers (10 miles) from this location, or any combination of such limitations).

2. Upon order of the CO, any time dose rates begin to rise rapidly (more than 2 rad/min):

a. Convert to implementation of paragraph 3(a) above.

b. Recall reconnaissance survey parties if possible.

4. MOVEMENT IN AND THROUGH FALLOUT AREAS

a. Route and radiological reconnaissance will be accomplished prior to moving a convoy through fallout areas.

b. Whenever possible, routes will be chosen so as to minimize average dose to unit personnel during movement.

c. Convoy will travel at maximum safe speed and no stops will be authorized in the contaminated area.

d. Disabled vehicles and equipment may be abandoned on order of the senior officer or NCO present. No patients or personnel will be abandoned. Location of abandoned vehicles or valuable equipment will be noted on a map so that such items may be retrieved when radiological decay makes this possible.

e. The lead vehicle of the convoy or each serial of the convoy will carry a monitor with a survey instrument and a map showing all reconnaissance data resulting from action in *a* above.

f. Continuous monitoring will be conducted.

g. Movement under extremely dusty conditions.

(1) Vehicles will space themselves in the column so as to minimize dust.

(2) Personnel riding in open vehicles (except drivers) will cover themselves with a poncho —head and all.

(3) Upon completing movement through the dusty contaminated area—

(*a*) Vehicles will be swept or brushed off.

(*b*) Personnel will remove ponchos and brush each other off.

(*c*) When time and the situation permit, vehicles will be washed and personnel will wash exposed skin surfaces.

(4) Whenever movement through or out of a fallout area has been completed, radiological data acquired will be promptly reported to the nearest headquarters for inclusion in CHEMRAD and CBROC information.

APPENDIX 2. FALLOUT SHELTER
(TO ANNEX G TO 9TH EVACUATION HOSPITAL FIELD SOP)

1. Application: Provisions of this appendix apply whenever the entire hospital including patients cannot be accommodated in existing shelter as provided for in II B 1b. (See page 71.)

2. As soon as it is determined that adequate fallout shelter is not available at a new hospital site, the Advance Party Commander will request immediate assistance from local Engineers in preparing fallout shelter.

3. When only a minimum of Engineer help is available, the following measures will permit fallout survival of unit personnal and patients:

a. Engineers will be requested to "slot doze" a trench 2.7 meters (9 feet) wide by at least 1.2 meter (4 feet) deep in 30 meter (100 foot) increments.

(1) 61 meters (200 feet) of such trenching will be dug for each 100 patients anticipated, plus at least 30 meters (100 feet) for unit personnel (depending upon the number to be accommodated in foxholes (b below).

(2) Trenching will be constructed so as to allow soil to accumulate along sides and at ends of trenches providing this does not add more than 5 minutes dozer time to each 30 meter (100 foot) trench. (In most soils, piles 61 centimeters (2 feet) high will normally accumulate along the sides and as much as 1.8 meter (6 feet) at the ends of the trench.)

(3) Drainage—Drainage of trenches will be accomplished by—

(a) Digging trenches on a 2–3 percent slope to facilitate drainage from the low end.

(b) "Crowning" the trench floor to allow drainage along sides of trench.

(c) Draining trenches from low end by constructing a sump or by ditching from low end of trenches to carry away water.

(d) Any other feasible method advised by the Engineers.

(4) Tentage.

(a) In each case, the CO will decide whether or not any tentage is to be erected over the slot-dozed trenches.

(b) When tents are erected over trenches, tent poles will be modified or elevated on chests or boxes.

(c) Roofs of tents erected over trenches will be covered with additional tent flies or tarps when possible.

b. The following shelters will be prepared by unit personnel (in priority):

(1) Prior to sleeping in the new site, unit personnel will dig two-man foxholes no less than 46 centimeters (18 inches) deep and large enough to lie in. Pup tents will be erected over these foxholes. This applies to the advance party as well as the main hospital unit.

(2) A shelter will be dug under the Headquarters tent large enough to accommodate the Hospital CO, XO, CBR O, CBR NCO, Opns Sgt, Switchboard Operator and communications equipment.

(3) Two-man foxholes will be prepared at each guard post and at the hospital ambulance entrance.

c. As time permits, all shelters will be improved by deepening, undercutting, covering open holes and trenches, sandbagging and any other measures designed to improve the protection offered and/or the comfort of occupants of the shelters.

4. When additional Engineer assistance is available (more than an absolute minimum), it will be used as directed by the CO (with advice from the CBR Officer) to improve the radiological protection offered and the comfort afforded shelter occupants.

5. If neither existing shelter or Engineer assistance is available—

a. Notify the next higher headquarters of the situation.

(1) Request permission to make limited adjustment in location to a new site where shelter exists (providing a satisfactory specific location has been determined).

(2) Or request permission to delay opening of hospital to receive patients until shelter for expected first 48-hour patient load can be prepared

by unit personnel. This patient shelter must be in addition to unit shelter prescribed in paragraph 3*b* above.

b. In the absence of permission to move to a new site, prepare basic fallout shelters with unit resources through a combination of foxholes, sandbagging, and judicious use of terrain irregularities.

c. Continue to improve shelters by all means available as time permits.

APPENDIX 3. THE RADIOLOGICAL OPERATIONS CENTER (ROC) (TO ANNEX G TO 9TH EVACUATION HOSPITAL FIELD SOP)

1. Function

The Radiological Operations Center (ROC) is a part of Hospital Headquarters which is responsible for all technical radiological operations during fallout. It will serve as a center for the collection and processing of radiological data to assist the CBR Officer in fulfilling his responsibilities to the Hospital Commander during fallout. Its specific functions are to furnish the Commander with information upon which to base decisions and to assist him in controlling the radiological situation with the hospital.

2. Activation

The Radiological Operations Center will be activated—

a. When the command "Prepare for Fallout" is given.

b. Upon order of the Hospital Commander or the CBR Officer.

3. Location

The ROC will be located in the Hospital Headquarters.

4. Composition

The ROC will be staffed by the following personnel:

a. The CBR Officer (who will command the center).

b. CBR NCO.

c. One Monitoring and Surveying Team (two persons).

5. Operation

The following activities will be carried on by the staff of the ROC:

a. *Prior to Fallout.* At command "Prepare for Fallout."—

(1) Establish the ROC.

(2) Notify monitoring and surveying teams to prepare for action.

(3) Obtain all possible information concerning the burst including: time of burst, yield, location, height of burst, anticipated fallout pattern, and ETA of fallout at hospital site. (Best probable source of information: nearest CBROC or Medical Section of a headquarters having a CBROC.)

(4) Initiate continuous monitoring.

(5) Give instructions and directions to the M & S Teams when they report.

b. *During Fallout.* (After dose rate of 1 rad/hr and rising has been read)—

(1) Continue to secure all possible information concerning the burst responsible for the fallout.

(2) Retain at least one IM–174A survey meter and one AN/PDR–27 monitoring meter, two IM–93 dosimeters and one PP–1578A charger at the ROC.

(3) Locate the two IM–93 dosimeters outside the ROC shelter 91 centimeters (3 feet) above the earth's surface in such a way that they can be reached for readings from time to time with a minimum of exposure to ROC personnel. Protect dosimeters from direct contamination (tie paper or condom over them).

(4) Distribute monitors and remaining radiac instruments throughout shelters as indicated by the situation.

(5) Direct the monitors to—

(a) Establish the protection factor of all shelters which can be reached without undue exposure. (Monitors divide instrument readings outside by the readings inside shelter to find protection factors.)

(b) Determine the uniformity of protection within each shelter.

(c) Report (a) and (b) above to ROC as soon as possible.

(6) Maintain a radiological situation map of suitable scale showing the fallout pattern and dose rates, whether this information has been received from reliable sources or estimated by the ROC staff.

(7) Maintain a record including at least the following:

(a) All information available concerning the burst believed to be responsible for the fallout.

(b) Date and time of onset of fallout.

(c) Dose rate, time readings at significant intervals as the fallout progresses. Intervals can be 1–2 minutes, 15 minutes or more depending upon the rapidity with which the radiological situation changes. Intensities should be unshielded dose rates determined by lifting the instrument outside shelter (or using a remote reading adaptation) or they should be read within the shelter and corrected for the shelter protection factor.

(d) Average total dose to date outside and inside shelter. If various shelters have significantly different protection factors, shelter dose estimates will be broken down by shelter if possible.

(8) Keep the Commanding Officer informed at all times concerning the radiological situation.

(9) As soon as the CBR Officer is convinced that ambient dose rates are dropping—

(a) The Hospital Commander will be notified that the peak has been passed.

(b) Word will be spread throughout the hospital that the peak has been passed.

(c) An estimate will be made as to the time and magnitude of the peak intensity.

(d) An estimate will be prepared of future intensities at various times, including a prediction as to when limited unshielded activity may be resumed or evacuation of the area may be possible. This information will be furnished the Commanding Officer and will be revised whenever better estimates are available.

c. *After Fallout.*

(1) Unless the hospital site is to be evacuated, a survey of the hospital area will be directed by the CBR Officer.

(a) Results will be recorded on a sketch map and reported to the Commanding Officer.

(b) "Hot spots" will be marked and avoided.

(2) Radiation exposures.

(a) *Unit.*

1. ROC personnel will prepare an estimate of average unit radiation dose within 12 hours after completion of the "acute" phase of fallout.

2. Where the protection afforded large groups of personnel in different shelters varied significantly, two or more average unit exposures may be reported. Groups to which each applied will be identified as clearly as possible (Unit EM in bivouac area; patients and personnel in patient

shelter system; personnel and patients in basement of red-brick building). If the CO desires, he may later request identification of one or more groups by names as accurately as the situation permits.

3. When the unit continues to receive significant radiation exposures subsequent to the "acute" phase (greater than 5 rad per day), a daily average unit exposure will be reported to the Hospital Commander.

(b) *Individual.*

1. Individual exposures of all personnel who were exposed to greater than the unit average dose will be estimated separately. This group will include monitors, surveyors, decontamination crews, late-arriving patients, and any personnel who left shelter to perform a special task.

2. Dose to any patient will be reported to the Registrar.

3. Names and estimated doses of each individual will be reported to the Hospital Commander within 12 hours after completion of the "acute" phase. Negative reports will be rendered.

4. If any individuals reported in *3* above are subjected to continued radiation doses immediately following the "acute" phase, a report of the estimated total dose of each will be rendered daily to the Hospital Commander by name.

(3) As long as the ROC is activated, it will control all monitoring and surveying activities including personnel and food and water monitoring.

(4) The order to resume operations outside shelter on any scale will not normally be given prior to the time intensities have dropped to 1 rad/hr unless ordered by higher headquarters.

6. Inactivation

a. The ROC will be inactivated when, in the opinion of the RDO (and with the approval of the Hospital Commander), the radiological situation no longer represents a direct hazard to life. Generally this will coincide with the abandonment of shelter.

b. After the inactivation of the ROC, the RDO will direct any further radiological activities from his regular office as an additional duty.

APPENDIX 4. FOOD AND WATER
(TO ANNEX G TO 9TH EVACUATION HOSPITAL FIELD SOP)

1. Purpose

This appendix outlines the policies for monitoring and consumption of food and water during and after radiological fallout.

2. Food

a. *During fallout* only C-type packaged rations provided in advance will be consumed.

b. *After the fallout*, packaged foods or unspoiled foods which have been well-covered during fallout can be consumed without radiological hazard.

c. *Subsequent ration issues.*

(1) Subsequent ration issues should have been cleared for consumption by supporting organizations prior to issue according to SOP. However, the CBR Officer will have unpackaged items of each ration issue "spot checked" for contamination for at least 1 week after fallout.

(2) Monitoring may be done in this manner—Remove food sample to the best fallout shelter available. If an AN/PDR–27 monitoring instrument indicates twice background dose rate when window or probe is passed approximately 15 centimeters (6 inches) from the surface, the food may be considered contaminated.

(3) If any food is considered contaminated—

(a) The Hospital Commander together with the CBR Officer will decide whether food should be decontaminated and consumed or disposed of.

(b) The class 1 Supply Point responsible for the issue will be notified.

3. Water

a. *During Fallout.* Water which was in covered containers before and during fallout (canteens, 5-gallon cans and water trailers) can be consumed without danger.

b. *Subsequent Water Issues.*

(1) Water supplied this unit from authorized water points should not be contaminated. However the CBR Officer will have water "spot checked" from time to time.

(2) Spot check of water may be accomplished in the following manner:

(a) In the best shelter available, check an empty 5-gallon can for contamination by passing the probe of an AN/PDR–27 within 15 centimeters (6 inches) of the surface of the can. Reading of twice current background or more indicates contamination.

(b) Fill an uncontaminated can with the water to be checked. In the same shelter as above, place probe of an AN/PDR–27 against the middle of the flat side of the can. A reading of twice current background or more indicates that the water is contaminated.

(3) If water is found to be contaminated—

(a) The CBR Officer will attempt to locate an uncontaminated source of water, with particular attention to ground waters (wells and springs).

(b) Extent of contamination will be reported to the Hospital Commanding Officer who will consider the CBR Officer's recommendation in deciding whether to allow the water to be consumed.

(c) When water is found to be contaminated and an uncontaminated source is not available—

1. Consumption of contaminated water will be limited to that necessary to sustain life and permit performance of duty. Canned juices and juicy canned foods may be substituted for water if available.

2. Samples of water will be dispatched to the supporting medical laboratory for radiological analysis.

3. The fact that radiologically contaminated water is being consumed will be reported to next higher headquarters.

APPENDIX 5. MONITORING AND SURVEYING TEAMS
(TO ANNEX G TO 9TH EVACUATION HOSPITAL FIELD SOP)

1. _____ Radiological Monitoring and Surveying Teams (M & S Teams) will be designated, trained, and equipped to perform M & S Team functions as an additional duty (at least one team per authorized monitoring or surveying radiac instrument).

2. Each team will consist of two persons: One instrument operator and one recorder-communicator, both trained in instrument operation.

3. At least 4 individuals trained as M & S alternates will be available at all times to fill vacancies on the M & S Teams.

4. Personnel designated for M & S Teams should come from those sections of the hospital whose activities are likely to cease or be greatly curtailed during fallout (motor pool and laundry).

5. Training.
   a. M & S personnel will be trained under the supervision of the CBR Officer.

   b. Specialized training (over and above unit radiological defense training) given to M & S personnel will total at least 30 hours of instruction other than on-the-job training.

   c. M & S personnel will have working knowledge of at least the following:

   (1) Use, maintenance, and operational checking of each type of radiac equipment authorized the unit.

   (2) How to evaluate the hazard represented by radiation measurements made in different ways at different times and under varying conditions.

   (3) Dose and intensity calculations such as dose rate at future times, total dose during various periods of time and under varying circumstances.

   (4) Means and methods for protection against fallout radiation.

   (5) The techniques of conducting, recording, and reporting monitoring and surveying operations.

   (6) Elementary nuclear weapons effects and characteristics of radiological fallout.

6. Operation.
   a. Monitors and Surveyors will report automatically to the CBR Officer or his designated representative with their equipment when the commands "Prepare for Fallout" or "Fallout" are passed through the unit. They will report at any other time upon order of the CBR Officer.

   b. During fallout or threat of fallout, they will continue to work under supervision of the CBR Officer until specifically released from their M & S duties by the CBR Officer.

   c. *During "acute" phase of fallout—*

   (1) One or more M & S Teams may be retained in the Radiological Operations Center to assist in its operation.

   (2) Other M & S personnel normally will be dispersed throughout the shelters as directed by the CBR Officer. Their functions during this period will include the following:

   (a) Advise personnel on radiological hazards and means of improving protection.

   (b) Advise the CBR Officer by any means of communication possible of any dangerous radiological conditions.

   (c) Continuously assess the radiological situation in their section of shelter to include—

   1. Effectiveness of cleanup of radioactive material.

   2. Protection factor of shelter.

   3. Current radiation intensities.

   4. Current average dose to personnel.

   5. Radiation exposure status of personnel who have performed tasks outside shelter.

   (d) Brief personnel who leave shelter, give them a dosimeter and upon their return, supervise their decontamination and read and record their exposure during the period outside shelter.

   d. *After "acute" phase of fallout—*

   (1) Teams equipped with IM–174A survey meters will perform surveys as assigned by the CBR Officer.

   (2) Teams equipped with AN/PDR–27 monitoring meter will perform monitoring tasks as assigned by the CBR Officer.

(3) M & S personnel may be—

(a) Employed by the CBR Officer to assist in recording radiological data, estimating dose to individuals and other clerical duties connected with the radiological history of the fallout event.

(b) Assigned to supervise decontamination operations and recommend methods for minimizing radiological hazards during their conduct.

(c) Called upon to conduct radiological road reconnaissance or to accompany motor convoys.

e. Before resuming their regular duties after being released by the CBR Officer, M & S personnel will clean or decontaminate instrument exteriors, and thoroughly check all radiac instruments (with special attention to battery checks) to assure that they are again ready for instant and prolonged use.

APPENDIX 6. RADIAC INSTRUMENTS
TO ANNEX G TO 9TH EVACUATION HOSPITAL FIELD SOP

1. Authorization.
    ..... IM-174A Radiac Meters (Survey Type).
    ..... IM-93 Dosimeters.
    .....PP-1578A/PD Chargers.
    ..... AN/PDR-27 Radiac Meters (G-M Type).

2. Radiac instruments will be turned in periodically for calibration as directed in current Army directives.

3. CBR NCO will have all instruments checked daily to assure that they are in good operating condition.

4. Defective instruments not locally repairable will be exchanged as soon as defect is noted.

5. Batteries. Replacement batteries will be ordered promptly every 6 months or whenever any set has had 100 hours of use. At least one complete set of replacement batteries will be kept on hand for each type of battery-operated instrument authorized.

6. Rate Meters IM-174A and AN/PDR-27.

    a. At least 1 IM-174A (survey meter) and 1 AN/PDR-27 (monitoring meter) will remain in Hospital Headquarters (ROC) at all times.

    b. Additional survey or monitoring instruments will be distributed as directed by the CBR Officer.

7. Tactical Dosimeters (IM-93 PLUS CHARGER, PP-1578A/PD).

    a. At least two IM-93 Dosimeters and one charger, PP-1578A/PD, will remain at Hospital Headquarters (ROC) at all times.

    b. Remaining dosimeters and chargers will remain in custody of monitoring and surveying team personnel except—

        (1) As otherwise directed by the CBR Officer.

        (2) Individuals leaving shelter for any reason will wear a dosimeter which will be charged before departure and read by a monitor upon return.

APPENDIX D

TRANSMISSION FACTORS FOR NUCLEAR RADIATION *

Environment shielding	Initial		Residual
	Neutrons	Gamma	
Armored carrier	0.7	0.7	0.6
Built-up city area (in open)	1.0	0.5	0.7
Foxholes	0.3	0.2	0.1
Frame house:			
First floor	1.0	0.9	0.5
Basement	0.5	0.3	0.1
Multistory buildings:			
Top floor	1.0	0.9	0.1
Intermediate floors	0.9	0.9	.02
Lower floor	0.9	0.5	0.1
Basement	0.5	0.3	.01
Shelter, Closed 91 cm. (3 ft)			
(earth cover)	0.05	0.02	0.005
Tanks:			
Light	0.3	0.2	0.2
Medium or heavy	0.3	0.1	0.1
Trucks:			
¼-ton	1.0	1.0	0.8
¾-ton	1.0	1.0	0.7
2½-ton	1.0	1.0	0.6
4–7-ton	1.0	1.0	0.5
Woods	1.0	1.0	0.8

* Inside Dose = Transmission factor times outside dose.

ACTIVE MATERIAL—Material, such as Plutonium and certain isotopes of uranium, which is capable of supporting a fission chain reaction. Active material is also called fissionable and nuclear material.

ABSORPTION—The process by which radiation imparts some or all of its energy to any material through which it passes.

ALPHA PARTICLE—(alpha radiation—a)—A particle emitted spontaneously from the nuclei of some radioactive elements, identical with the helium nucleus, having two protons and two neutrons, a mass of about 4 units and an electric charge of 2 positive units.

ATOM—The smallest particle of an element that still retains the characteristics of that element and which is capable of entering into a chemical reaction.

ATOMIC MASS UNIT (amu)—1/12 of the mass of one neutral atom of ^{12}C.

ATOMIC NUMBER (Z)—Number of orbital electrons in a neutral atom, or the electric charge on the nucleus of an atom, or the number of protons in the atomic nucleus.

ATOMIC WEAPONS—*See* nuclear weapon.

ATOMIC WEIGHT (A)—The relative weight of an atom of an element compared with the weight of 1 atom of carbon taken as 12. A multiple of 1/12 of the weight of an atom of carbon.

ATTENUATION—The process by which a beam of radiation is reduced in intensity when passing through some material. It is the combination of absorption and scattering processes.

BACKGROUND RADIATION—Nuclear or ionizing radiations arising from within the body and from the surroundings to which individuals are always exposed. The main sources of natural background radiation are potassium–40 in the body, potassium–40 and thorium, uranium, and their decay products (including radium) present in rocks, and cosmic rays.

BETA PARTICLE (β)—A negatively or positively (positron) charged particle having a mass equal to the electron and emitted spontaneously from the nuclei of certain radioactive elements.

BIOLOGICAL HALF-TIME—The time required for the amount of a specified element which has entered the body (or a particular organ) to be decreased to half of its initial value as a result of natural, biological elimination processes.

CHAIN REACTION—A process in which some of the products of a step in the process are instrumental in causing a continuation or magnification of the process. Specifically, a fission chain reaction in active material is continued or magnified by the neutrons which are one of the products of fission itself.

CONTAMINATION—The deposit of radioactive material on the surfaces of structures, areas, objects or personnel, following a nuclear explosion.

CRITICAL MASS—The minimum mass of a fissionable material that will just maintain a fission chain reaction under precisely specified conditions, such as the nature of the material and its purity, the nature and thickness of the tamper (or neutron reflector), the density (or compression), and the physical shape (or geometry). For an explosion to occur, the system must be supercritical; i.e., the mass of material must exceed the critical mass under the existing conditions.

CRITICAL ORGAN—That part of the body that is most susceptible to radiation damage under the specific conditions considered; determined by the following criteria: (1) Organ that concentrates greatest amount of radioactive material; (2) Indispensability of the organ to overall well-being of body; (3) The organ damaged by entry of radionuclide into body; (4) The radiosensitivity of the organ.

CURIE—A unit of radioactivity. That quantity of a radioactive nuclide disintegrating at the rate of 3.7×10^{10} atoms per second.

DECAY (OR RADIOACTIVE DECAY)—The decrease in activity of any radioactive material with the passage of time, due to the spontaneous emission of α, β, or γ radiation from the nuclei of unstable atoms.

DECAY PRODUCT (DAUGHTER PRODUCT)—The daughter nuclide resulting from the radioactive disintegration of a radionuclide or series of radionuclides. A decay product may be either stable or radioactive.

DECONTAMINATION—The reduction or removal of contaminating radioactive material from a structure, or an object or person. Decontamination may be accomplished by (1) treating the surface so as to remove or decrease the contamination; (2) letting the material stand so that the radioactivity is decreased as a result of natural decay; and (3) covering the contamination so as to attenuate the radiation emitted.

DEUTERIUM (D OR ²H)—A heavy, stable isotope of hydrogen having 1 proton and 1 neutron in the nucleus.

DISINTEGRATION—Process of spontaneous breakdown of a nucleus of an atom resulting in the emission of a particle and/or a photon.

DOSE—The amount of ionizing radiation energy absorbed per unit mass of irradiated material at a specific location, such as a part of the human body. Measured in roentgens, rep, rem, and rad.

DOSE RATE—The amount of ionizing (or nuclear) radiation received per unit time; usually expressed in rad/hr.

DOSIMETER—An instrument for measuring and registering total accumulated exposure to ionizing radiation.

ECCHYMOSIS—An extravasation of blood; a discoloration of the skin caused by the extravasation of blood.

ELECTRON—A particle of very small mass, carrying a unit negative or positive charge. Negative electrons surround the nucleus in all neutral atoms. Their number is equal to the positive charges (protons) in the nucleus.

ELECTRON VOLT—A unit of energy equivalent to the amount of energy gained by an electron passing through a potential difference of 1 volt.
  a. Kev for thousand or Kilo electron volts.
  b. Mev for million electron volts.
  c. Bev for billion electron volts.

ENERGY—The ability to do work. Energy (E) is the force (f) acting on a body to produce motion, multiplied by the distance (S) through which the force acts and the cosine of the angle (θ) between the direction of force and the direction of motion. $E = fS \cos \theta$. *Potential energy* is energy due to relative position, e.g., and elevated weight. *Kinetic energy* is energy due to motion—a speeding auto or electron. Energy is measured in ergs, joules, ev, Mev, etc.

ERYTHEMA—An abnormal redness of the skin caused by a variety of agents, including ionizing radiations.

EXPLOSIVE SYSTEM—That portion of a nuclear weapon which transforms the nuclear system from a subcritical to a supercritical state.

FALLOUT—The radioactive debris, usually from a nuclear detonation, which is deposited on the surface after having been airborne. Local (or early) fallout is defined, somewhat arbitrarily, as those particles which reach the earth within 24 hours after a nuclear explosion. Worldwide (or Delayed) fallout consists of the smaller particles which ascend into the upper troposphere and into the stratosphere and are carried by winds to all parts of the earth. The worldwide fallout is brought to earth, mainly by rain and snow, over extended periods ranging from months to years.

FISSION—The process whereby the nucleus of a particular heavy element splits (generally) into 2 nuclei of lighter elements with the release of substantial amounts of energy. The fissionable materials that are most frequently used in nuclear weapons are 235 uranium and 239 plutonium.

FISSION PRODUCTS—A general term for the complex mixture of substances produced as a result of nuclear fission. A distinction should be made between these and the direct fission products or fission fragments. Something like 80 different fission fragments result from roughly 40 different modes of fission of a given nuclear species (e.g., 235 uranium or 239 plutonium). The fission fragments, being radioactive, immediately begin to decay, forming additional (daughter) products, with the result that the complex mixture of fission products so formed contains about 200 different isotopes of 37 elements.

FISSIONABLE MATERIAL—*See* **active material.**

FUSION—The process whereby the nuclei of light elements, especially those of the isotopes of hydrogen (deuterium and tritium), combine to form the nucleus of a heavier element with the release of substantial amounts of energy.

GAMMA RAY (γ)—High frequency (short wave length) electromagnetic radiation emitted by the nucleus of an atom.

GEIGER-MUELLER (G-M) TUBE—A gas-filled tube operated with a high voltage such that a discharge is triggered by single ionizing event. Used in instruments measuring low levels of radiation.

GRANULOCYTE—Any cell containing granules, especially a leukocyte (white blood cell) containing neutrophilic, basophilic, or eosinophilic granules in its cytoplasm.

GROUND ZERO (GZ)—The point on the earth's surface at which, above which, or below which a nuclear detonation has actually occurred or will occur.

GUN-TYPE WEAPON (OR GUN-ASSEMBLY WEAPON)—A device in which two or more pieces of fissionable material, each in a subcritical state, are brought together very rapidly so as to form a supercritical mass which can explode as the result of a rapidly expanding fission chain reaction.

HALF-LIFE—The time required for the activity of a given radioactive isotope to decrease to half of its initial value due to radioactive decay. The half-life is a characteristic property of each radioactive isotope and is independent of its amount or condition. The effective half-life of a given isotope is the time which the quantity in the body will decrease to half as a result of both radioactive decay and biological elimination.

HALF-VALUE LAYER (HVL)—Amount of shielding material necessary to reduce the intensity of radiation by a factor of 2.

HYDROGEN BOMB—*See* **thermonuclear weapons.**

IMPLOSION-TYPE WEAPON (IMPLOSION WEAPON)—A device in which a quantity of fissionable material, in a subcritical state, has its volume suddenly decreased by compression so that it becomes supercritical and explodes. The compression is achieved by means of a spherical arrangement of specially fabricated shapes of ordinary high explosive which produce an inwardly directed implosion wave. The fissionable material, being at the center of the sphere, is thereby compressed to a supercritical state.

INDUCED RADIOACTIVITY—Radioactivity produced in certain materials as a result of nuclear reactions, particularly the capture of neutrons, which are accompanied by the formation of unstable (radioactive) nuclei.

INITIAL RADIATION—Nuclear radiation (essentially neutrons and gamma rays) emitted from the fireball and the cloud column during the first minute after a nuclear detonation.

ION—An atom or molecule that has lost or gained one or more electrons by ionization; it becomes electrically charged.

IONIZATION—The process whereby energy is acquired by a neutral atom or molecule resulting in the ejection of an orbital electron and producing two charged particles, i.e., an ion pair.

IONIZATION (ION) CHAMBER—An instrument that detects and measures ionizing radiation by observing the electrical current created when radiation ionizes gas in the chamber, making it a conductor of electricity.

IONIZING RADIATION—Electromagnetic radiation (X or γ photons) or corpuscular radiation (α particles, β particles, negatrons, positrons, protons, neutrons, and heavy particles) capable of producing ions by direct or indirect processes.

ISOTOPES—Atoms of the same element having identical chemical properties, but differing in their atomic masses (due to different numbers of neutrons in their respective nuclei).

KILOTON (KT)—Refers to the energy release in the explosion of 1,000 tons of TNT where 1 ton equals 2,000 pounds.

LYMPHOCYTE—A variety of white corpuscle (blood cell) which arises in the reticular tissue of the lymph glands and in other tissue. The nucleus is single and large and is surrounded by protoplasm which is generally described as nongranular.

MASS—The material equivalent of energy—different from weight in that it neither increases nor decreases with gravitational force.

MASS NUMBER (A)—The number of nucleons (neutrons and protons) in the nucleus of an atom.

MEGATON (MT)—Refers to the energy release in the explosion of a million tons of TNT.

MOLECULE—A group of atoms held together by chemical forces. The atoms in the molecule may be identical, H_2, or different, H_2O.

NEUTRON—Elementary nuclear particle with a mass approximately equal to that of a hydrogen atom and electrically neutral.

NONEFFECTIVE—As applied to an individual, one who cannot perform his assigned mission or task.

NUCLEAR MATERIAL—*See* **active material.**

NUCLEAR RADIATION—Any electromagnetic waves or nuclear particles emitted from the nucleus of an atom.

NUCLEAR WEAPON (ATOMIC BOMB)—A general name given to any weapon in which the explosion results from the energy released by reactions involving atomic nuclei, either fission or fusion, or both. Thus, the A- (or atomic) bomb and the H- (or hydrogen) bomb are both nuclear weapons. It would be equally true to call them atomic weapons, since it is the energy of the atomic nuclei that is involved in each case. However, it has become more or less customary, although it is not strictly accurate, to refer to weapons in which all the energy results from fission as A-bombs or atomic bombs. To make a distinction, those weapons in which part, at least, of the energy results from *thermonuclear* (fusion) reactions among the isotopes of hydro-

gen have been called H-bombs or hydrogen bombs.

NUCLEON—A constituent of the atomic nucleus; e.g., a proton or neutron.

NUCLEUS—The heavy central part of an atom in which most of the mass and the total positive electric charge is concentrated.

NUCLIDE—A general term referring to all nuclear species, both stable and unstable, of the chemical elements, as distinguished from the two or more nuclear species of a single chemical element which are called "isotopes."

OVERPRESSURE—The transient pressure, usually expressed in pounds per square inch (psi), exceeding existing atmospheric pressure and manifested in the shock or blast wave from an explosion.

PAIR PRODUCTION—The process whereby a γ ray or X-ray photon, with energy in excess of 1.02 Mev, in passing near the nucleus of an atom is converted into a positive electron and negative electron. As a result, the photon ceases to exist.

PEAK OVERPRESSURE—The highest overpressure resulting from the blast wave. Peak overpressures near the fireball of a nuclear explosion are very high, but drop off rapidly as the blast wave travels along the ground outward from ground zero.

PETECHIAE—Small, pinpoint, nonraised, round purplish-red spots caused by intradermal or submucous hemorrhage, which later turn blue or yellow.

PHOTOELECTRIC EFFECT—A process by which a photon ejects an electron from an atom. All the energy of the photon is absorbed in ejecting the electron and in imparting kinetic energy to it. As a result, the photon ceases to exist.

PHOTON—A quantity of electromagnetic energy whose value in ergs is the product of its frequency in cycles per second and Planck's constant.

POSITRON—A positively charged electron.

PROTON (p)—An elementary nuclear particle with a positive electric charge equal numerically to the charge of the electron and having a mass of 1.00759 AMU.

PURPURA—A bleeding or hemorrhagic condition characterized by the presence of confluent petechiae or confluent ecchymoses over any part of the body.

RAD—Radiation absorbed dose. The basic unit of absorbed dose of ionizing radiation. One rad is equal to the absorption of 100 ergs of radiation energy per gram of matter. For training and operational aspects of nuclear warfare, the *rad* is the official, authorized unit for use throughout the Army.

RADIATION—The propagation of energy through matter or space in the form of waves. In nuclear physics the term has been extended to include fast moving particles (alpha and beta particles, free neutrons, etc.).

RADIOACTIVITY—Process whereby certain nuclides undergo spontaneous disintegration in which energy is liberated, generally resulting in the formation of new nuclides. The process is accompanied by the emission of one or more types of radiation, such as alpha particles and gamma photons.

RANGE (of α or β particles)—The distance a particle will penetrate a given material before all of its ionizing power is spent.

RBE (RELATIVE BIOLOGICAL EFFECTIVENESS)—The RBE is a factor which is used to compare the biological effectiveness of absorbed radiation doses (i.e., rad) of different types of ionizing radiation. More specifically, it is the ratio of an absorbed dose of X-rays or γ rays to the absorbed dose of a certain particulate radiation or the radiation under investigation required to produce an identical biological effect in a particular experimental organism or tissue.

REM (ROENTGEN EQUIVALENT MAN)—A unit of absorbed dose in biological matter. It is equal to the absorbed dose in rads multiplied by the RBE of the radiation.

RESIDUAL NUCLEAR RADIATION—Nuclear radiation, chiefly beta particles and gamma rays, which persist for some time following a nuclear explosion. The radiation is emitted mainly by the fission products and other bomb residue in the fallout, and to some extent by earth and water constituents and other materials in which radioactivity has been induced by the capture of neutrons.

ROENTGEN (r)—An exposure dose of X or γ radiation such that the associated corpuscular emission (i.e., electrons) per 0.001293 grams of air produces, in air, ions carrying 1 esu of electricity of either sign.

SCATTERING—Change of direction of subatomic particles or photons as a result of a collision or interaction.

SECONDARY BLAST INJURIES—Those injuries sustained from the indirect blast effects, such as from falling rubble from a collapsed building or from missiles (debris or objects) which have been picked up by the winds generated and hurled against an individual. Also includes injuries resulting from individuals being hurled against stationary objects. (Sometimes referred to as tertiary effect.)

SUPERCRITICAL—The term applied to fissionable material which has been altered from the critical state, (by a change in its mass, density, or shape or by tamping) to a condition in which the neutrons produced inside the material increase rapidly and uncontrollably to produce a nuclear explosion. The number of fissions increase geometrically, and the neutrons produced thereby will sustain an increasing or multiplying chain reaction.

TENTH-VALUE LAYER (TVL)—Amount of shielding material required to reduce radiation intensity by a factor of 10.

THERMAL RADIATION—Electromagnetic radiation emitted from the fireball as a consequence of its very high temperature; it consists essentially of ultraviolet, visible, and infrared radiation.

THERMONUCLEAR (THERMONUCLEAR WEAPONS)—An adjective referring to the process (or processes) in which very high temperatures are used to bring about the fusion of light nuclei, such as those of the hydrogen isotopes (deuterium and tritium), with the accompanying liberation of energy. A thermonuclear bomb is a weapon in which part of the explosion energy results from thermonuclear fusion reactions. The high temperatures required may be obtained by means of a fission explosion.

TRITIUM (T OR ³H)—A radioactive isotope of hydrogen having 1 proton and 2 neutrons in the nucleus.

WEAPON EFFECTS—The damage or casualty producing agents, specifically blast, thermal radiation, and nuclear radiation, resulting from a nuclear explosion.

WEAPONS SYSTEM—The combination of the weapon, the fire control system, and the carrier.

X-RAYS—Penetrating electromagnetic radiation having wave lengths shorter than those of visible light. They are usually produced by bombarding a metallic target with fast electrons in a vacuum.

YIELD (OR ENERGY YIELD)—The total effective energy released in a nuclear (or atomic) explosion. It is usually expressed in terms of the equivalent tonnage of TNT required to produce the same energy release in an explosion.

By Order of the Secretary of the Army:

W. C. WESTMORELAND,
General, United States Army,
Chief of Staff.

Official:
KENNETH G. WICKHAM,
Major General, United States Army,
The Adjutant General.

Distribution:
Active Army:

DCSPER (2)	ARADCOM (2)
ACSI (2)	ARADCOM Rgn (1)
DCSOPS (2)	USACDC (2)
ACSFOR (2)	USAMC (2)
CORC (2)	Armies (1)
CRD (1)	Corps (1)
COA (1)	Div (1)
CINFO (1)	LOGCOMD (1)
TIG (1)	Bde (1)
TJAGSA (1)	Regt (1)
CNGB (2)	Gp (1)
TSG (30)	Gen Hosp (10)
USCONARC (5)	Army Hosp (5)
Br Svc Sch (1) except	All TOE 8—Units (3)
MFSS (100)	

NG: State AG (3); units—same as active Army, except allowance is one (1) copy per unit.
USAR: Same as active Army, except allowance is one (1) copy per unit. For explanation of abbreviations used, see AR 320–50.

☆ U.S. GOVERNMENT PRINTING OFFICE: 1969 0-349-756